Colonic Irrigation Hydrotherapy and Colon Cleanses

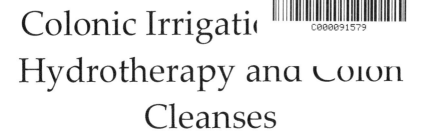

Includes facts, diet, health benefits, weight loss, cost, kits, procedures, natural cleansing, therapists and colon care

The Complete Guide

Donna Green

Published by ROC Publishing 2013

Foreword

The modern world, with its conveniences and advances is also a sea of toxic chemicals. No matter where we are, if we are breathing the air around us, drinking the water, or even eating "safe" food from the grocery shelves, we are ingesting unnatural substances.

Pesticides make their way into the ground water, while municipal systems are heavily laced with pharmaceuticals. Meats are injected with growth hormones. The grain in a simple loaf of bread may have been genetically modified, and it is certainly packed with gluten.

Our least expensive dietary choices are filled with processed sugars, food dyes, preservatives, and staggering amounts of sodium — the list is frightening and almost endless.

This is what we're asking our digestive systems to process. How is the body supposed to draw proper nutrition from this poisonous soup and, at the same time, protect us from harm? It is, at best, a tall order.

With increasing awareness, more and more people are turning to organic produce, opting for a more plant-based diet, eschewing artificial sweeteners, and trying to counteract the effects of all this "modernity" on their systems.

As added insult, however, while modern "convenience" is killing us, modern medicine labels natural and alternative treatments as ineffective at best, and at worst harmful and dangerous. Yet, many of these therapies, including colonic hydrotherapy, have literally been around for centuries.

If a big pharmaceutical company developed a new colonic hydrotherapy treatment, it might be dizzying to see how fast an approach to good health that is currently derided might be lauded in the name of greater profits.

Colon cleansing or irrigation works on the simple principle that our digestive tract, under siege from agents in our environment, must be cleaned out periodically. Otherwise, the accumulation of toxins leads to chronic inflammation, which modern medicine does recognize as a fertile breeding ground for a host of diseases.

If you are reading this book, you are at least curious about what colonic hydrotherapy involves. The text will attempt to answer that question and more, helping you to understand the workings of the digestive system, how it can be supported naturally, and how and when additional supportive care like colonic irrigation might be necessary.

I am not a medical doctor, and this text is not to be taken as medical advice. What I offer here is rather a detailed overview of an alternative therapy that can and does change lives when performed in a proper setting by a trained professional, or carried out in the privacy of your home with safe, viable products.

It is important to never adopt any health-based procedure without conducting complete and thorough research. Colonic irrigation is, for many people, a frightening thing to even think about or something that seems far too private and personal to be up for discussion.

Whether you opt for the help of a registered professional, or choose to pursue colon cleansing on another level, there are compelling arguments to be made for the need to support our digestive system more aggressively to counteract the effects of the toxins that assault us from every direction.

By the end of this book, you should be able to make an informed decision about what is right for you and your health.

With colonic hydrotherapy in its current state of evolution, there are far more benefits that you may realize — and far fewer risks.

The final decision, however, as with all things health-related, should be yours and yours alone.

Never give in to pressure from any one to have any treatment or medical procedure until you are 100% comfortable with the idea of proceeding and understand everything that is involved and all possible consequences.

Achieving that goal on your behalf is the point of this book.

Acknowledgements

I am so grateful to my partner for first introducing me to the world of colonics. It was an unforgettable experience and the journey has impacted on my life on many levels.

Thank you for all your support in writing this book – I love you from the bottom of my heart.

Table of Contents

Clarification of Terms

The text of this book uses the terms "irrigation" and "hydrotherapy" interchangeably. In order to avoid confusion, I want to clarify these terms, which are essentially identical, along with the more generic reference "cleanse."

Colon irrigation

"Colonic irrigation is also known as hydrotherapy of the colon, high colonic, entero-lavage, or simply colonic. It is the process of cleansing the colon by passing several gallons of water through it with the use of special equipment. It is similar to an enema but treats the whole colon, not just the lower bowel. This has the effect of flushing out impacted fecal matter, toxins, mucous, and even parasites, that often build up over the passage of time. It is a procedure that should only be undertaken by a qualified practitioner." *(Gale Encyclopedia of Medicine. Copyright 2008 The Gale Group, Inc. All rights reserved.)*

Colon hydrotherapy

[Colon hydrotherapy] is an extended and more complete form of an enema as well as a method of removing waste from the large intestine without using drugs. Colon hydrotherapy is used to treat constipation or impaction, as preparation for diagnostic studies of the large intestine (barium enema, sigmoidoscopy, or colonoscopy), and as preparation before or after surgery. The procedure is also used for bowel training for paraplegics or tetraplegics, those with arthritis, and patients who have suspected autointoxication or intestinal toxemia. *(Mosby's Medical Dictionary, 8th edition. © 2009, Elsevier.)*

Colon cleanse

A generic term for various types of enema, which are claimed to balance body chemistry, eliminate waste, and restore proper tissue and organ function. *(Segen's Medical Dictionary. © 2012 Farlex, Inc. All rights reserved.)*

For the proponents of the practice of colonic irrigation or colonic hydrotherapy — and there are many — the procedure is regarded as a safe and effective means to remove harmful debris from the large intestine.

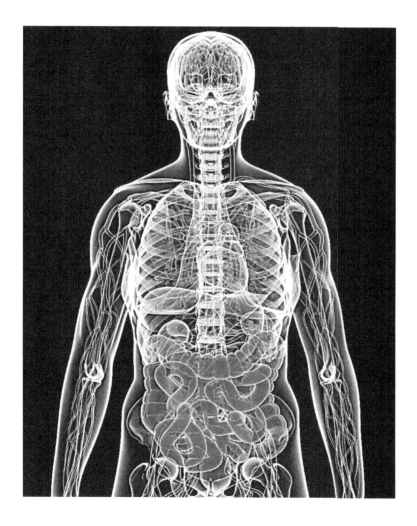

No drugs are used, only temperature-controlled, filtered water to soften and to remove accumulated waste via the natural muscle movement called peristalsis.

Colonic therapy is not a new idea. Its origins are much older than most people realize, and the techniques have improved steadily from simple enemas to the sophisticated devices used in registered therapeutic settings today.

There are also many products available for home use, and growing numbers of people report significant improvement in their health after turning to some form of this centuries old cleansing process.

History of Colonic Irrigation

The first recorded use of enemas to improve health can be traced to the ancient Egyptians. The Ebers Papyrus, housed in the Royal Museum of Berlin, and dating to the 14th century BC contains enema-based remedies for more than 20 complaints of the stomach and intestines.

Babylonian and Assyrian tablets from 600 BC include similar references, and both the Greeks and Romans considered enemas as viable fever therapy and a cure for worms. The third century Essene Gospel contains the following passage:

"The uncleanness within is greater than the uncleanness without. And he who cleanses himself without, but within remains unclean, is like a tomb that outward is painted fair, but is within full of all manner of horrible uncleanness and abominations."

By the Middle Ages, the wealthy regarded the use of enemas as a trendy vogue. The 17th century is referred to as the "age of the enema," with fashionable Parisians taking three or four treatments a day.

Syringes used to perform the procedure were elaborate and often made of copper or porcelain and inlaid with mother of pearl and silver. Of course, colonic cleansing practices have always endured droll asides. In Spain, for instance, enemas were known as "playing the bagpipes."

The use of enemas reached its peak in the late 17th and early 18th centuries before dwindling in the late 19th and early 20th centuries.

The development of effective laxatives and other commercial drugs provided less invasive alternatives to enemas and to any of the other colon cleansing apparatus that had been developed.

With the publication of the book "Colonic Irrigation" by Dr. W. Kerr Russell in 1932, the more modern method of hydrotherapy began to gain notice, however.

The intent of the treatment was to remove abnormal mucus from the walls of the bowel as well as to empty the bowel tract. Russell argued that as a result, both the tone of the colonic muscle and the blood supply in the organ were improved.

Colonic hydrotherapy continued to evolve in sophistication throughout the 1940s and 1950s, only to disappear again in the 1960s and 1970s.

Many of the conditions once treated with hydrotherapy were addressed with Fleet enemas, prescription laxatives, and in severe cases the colostomy.

Today, however, alternative health practitioners are once again turning to colon cleansing as a method for detoxification and weight loss.

The state of the modern diet underlies this trend. Chemicals and other contaminants in our food, and the alarming rise of autoimmune diseases further bolster evidence of the therapy's efficacy.

Benefits of Colonic Irrigation

There are many reputed benefits of colonic irrigation, including, but not limited to:

- Improved bowel regularity, especially for those patients suffering from irritable bowel syndrome or chronic constipation.

- Better digestion and thus improved absorption of nutrients.

- A boosting of the immune system.

- Alkalization of the body leading to better sleep, more youthful skin, improved energy, higher resistance to disease, relief from arthritis, protection against osteoporosis, and sharper mental clarity.

- An overall improvement in mood with less depression and anxiety.

- Effective weight loss and body shaping.

In addition, colonic irrigation helps to hydrate the body. Chronic dehydration is a leading contributor to a host of modern ills including chronic fatigue syndrome, joint pain, and weight gain.

Understanding the Digestive System

How can colonic cleansing achieve such wide ranging results? It does so by boosting the functioning of the digestive system, which is responsible for efficiently feeding all parts of the body. In addition to being subject to physical defects, our digestion can also be deeply affected by stress in our lives.

Most of us have only the most cursory understanding of how the human digestive system works, and we tend to think everything begins in the stomach. That is far from the case.

DIGESTIVE SYSTEM

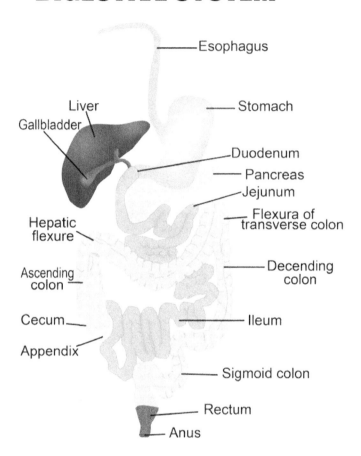

The Mouth

The first stage of breaking down food for utilization by the body occurs in the mouth. This involves both the action of chewing and the production of saliva to facilitate swallowing.

With the action of swallowing, food begins to move down the pharynx or throat before entering the esophagus on its way downward through the body to the stomach.

Esophagus and Stomach

The muscular tube of the esophagus links the pharynx to the stomach. Muscular contractions called peristalsis serve to move food toward the lower esophageal sphincter.

This round muscle sits in an area known as the "zone of high pressure." Essentially the sphincter works as a valve for the purpose of preventing food from changing direction and moving back up the tube.

The stomach, for its parts, is a muscular sac with strong walls that grind and mix the food with powerful secretions of acid and enzymes. When this process is complete, the digested material has reached the consistency of a liquid paste.

Small Intestine

In this state of digestion, food then enters the small intestine, an organ comprised of three parts: the duodenum, the jejunum, and the ileum. If the small intestine were spread out, it would look like a 20-foot (6.1 meters) long tube.

Three organs aid the small intestine: the pancreas, liver, and gallbladder. Enzymes from the pancreas work to break down fat, protein, and carbohydrates, while the liver secretes bile to cleanse the nutrient-rich blood coming away from the small intestine.

Bile is stored in the gallbladder. During a meal, contractions in the gallbladder dispatch bile to the small intestine.

When all nutrients have been removed from the food in the small intestine, the leftover material moves on to the large intestine or colon.

Large Intestine or Colon

The colon is also a muscular tube, some 5-6 feet (1.5 – 1.8 meters) in length. It connects the cecum to the rectum and is comprised of the ascending colon (right), the transverse colon (across), the descending colon (left), and the "s" shaped sigmoid colon.

Peristalsis moves waste or stool through the colon where it is stored in the sigmoid colon just above the rectum. It is held there until a mass movement empties the material once or twice a day (under optimal circumstances.) Typically it takes 36 hours for stool to move through the colon. The material is made up of bacteria and food debris.

Rectum

The 8-inch (20.3 cm) long rectum connects the colon to the anus. It serves to receive stool and to send a signal to the brain when the chamber is filled and ready for evacuation.

At that time, sphincter muscles relax and the rectum expels the material through a series of contractions.

Anus

The final portion of the digestive tract, the anus, is composed of the muscles of the pelvic floor, and the internal and external anal sphincter muscles.

The pelvic floor muscles form an angle between the rectum and anus and prevent the improper evacuation of the accumulated material.

The underlying theory of colonic irrigation is the idea of "autointoxification." The belief is that the improper cleansing of waste material in the colon causes the left over debris to rot, creating a breeding ground ripe for infection and inflammation. From these conditions, a number of serious and life-altering health issues can evolve.

Diseases of the Colon

Disease of the colon can range from the presence of cancerous masses to the uncomfortable symptoms of Irritable Bowel Syndrome. Poor digestion can necessitate surgery, or cause a person to radically alter both their diet and lifestyle.

(Some of the major health problems associated with the colon are discussed below. Please note that this is not an all-inclusive list, but only the most commonly seen conditions.)

Polyps

Polyps are the most common non-cancerous growths to be found on the lining of the colon. They are small balls of abnormal cells attached to stalks. Typically the masses are 2 mm to 5 cm or more in diameter.

It is important to determine the nature of the cells forming the polyp to accurately judge the risk of cancer developing. Metaplastic polyps do not present a danger, but adenomatous polyps can become malignant.

Even in a healthy colon, about 10% of the cells present exhibit pronounced abnormality. In most cases, however, these cells die a "pre-programmed" death via the process of apoplosis and fall harmlessly into the lumen or bowel cavity.

If a polyp grows to a diameter of 2 cm bleeding from the anus will usually begin, with evidence visible in underwear, on toilet paper, or via black or red-streaked stools.

Either diarrhea or constipation may be present for more than a week at a time. The diarrhea will be profuse and watery, which can lead to muscle weakness due to potassium deficiency. Severe abdominal pain is possible. Polyps can be detected during a colonoscopy, which examines the entire length of the bowel. The growths may be removed during that procedure while the patient is already sedated.

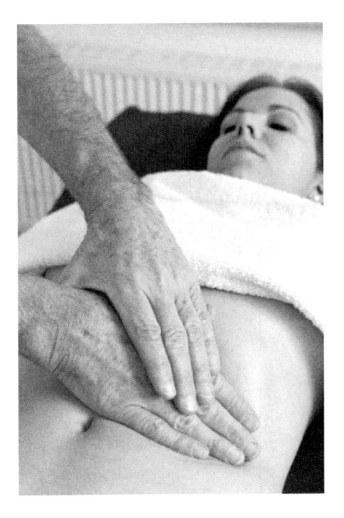

Other diagnostic procedures include a sigmoidoscopy (which examines the last third of the colon), a barium enema, and a digital examination.

Although dietary changes are not considered effective by many experts, the risk of polyps has been found to be significantly lower in non-smokers, people who do not consume fatty foods and maintain a normal weight, individuals that exercise regularly, and those who do not drink.

Other Benign Growths

Benign masses in the colon include neoplasm or tumors that do not recur after removal. These growths are contained clumps of tissue that serve no purpose and do not spread, but they do compromise the health of surrounding tissue. They grow more slowly, and are less likely to cause problems.

Any mass of this type can also be detected during a colonoscopy and will either be removed or biopsied during the procedure.

Diverticulitis

Diverticulitis is caused by eating a diet low in fiber. A diverticuli is a ruptured spot in the colon that causes an infection in adjacent tissue.

The subsequent pressure then leads to sacs that bulge or push outward from the colon. A single site is called a diverticulum, while multiple affected areas are diverticuli.

These ruptures and bulges can occur anywhere in the colon, but typically are located toward the end of the sigmoid.

Symptoms of their presence include bleeding, constipation, abdominal cramping, and potentially colon obstruction. When infection sets in, the abdomen may be tender and painful, and the individual may run a fever.

Other symptoms can include vomiting, bloating, abnormal urination (frequent and/or painful), and rectal bleeding.

Diverticulitis is most common in the developed nations of the world, and less prevalent in Africa and Asia. People younger than 40 years of age rarely develop the condition, but 15% of people age 60 or more in the United States suffer from the problem.

Recommended courses of treatment vary with the severity of and number of acute episodes. If the episode is mild, a liquid or low fiber diet in combination with a course of antibiotics may be recommended.

Individuals at high risk of infection or repeated episodes may face surgery to have the diseased portion of the intestine removed. In very severe cases, a temporary colostomy may be necessary until the intestine has properly healed.

Ulcerative Colitis

Ulcerative colitis is a form of inflammatory bowel disease characterized by the presence of open sores or ulcers causing constant diarrhea mixed with blood. The condition is often confused with both Crohn's Disease and Irritable Bowel Syndrome.

Ulcerative colitis is, however, an intermittent disease. Patients may go for extended periods during which they suffer no symptoms whatsoever.

The incidence rate is about 1 in 20 people per 100,000 on an annual basis with a greater number of cases in the developed world (especially in affluent nations.)

There is no known cause for ulcerative colitis although a genetic susceptibility is strongly assumed. An episode can be triggered by environmental factors, but the condition is not believed to be caused by diet.

Modifications in diet can, however, reduce the degree of discomfort experienced. Typical treatment is with anti-inflammatory medications.

Crohn's Disease

Crohn's Disease (Chrohn's Syndrome or Regional Enteritis) is also an inflammatory condition of the bowel, but may actually affect any part of the gastrointestinal tract from the mouth to the anus.

The disease is responsible for a broad range of symptoms including, but not limited to, pain in the abdomen, diarrhea (often bloody), vomiting (which may be continuous), and weight loss.

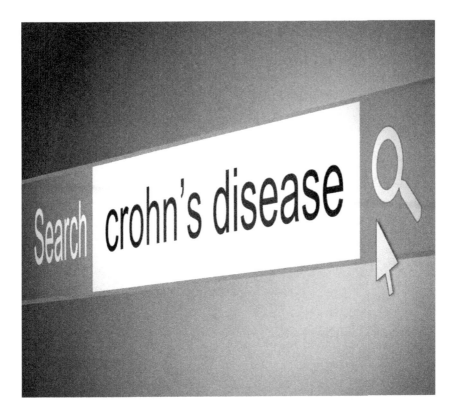

Crohn's is caused by an interaction of multiple factors including environmental, immunological, and bacterial.

There is a genetic susceptibility and this is a chronic inflammatory disease in which the body's immune system begins to attack the GI tract.

There is no cure, and remissions are never certain. The best approach endorsed by conventional medicine is to use a combination of medication with lifestyle and dietary changes.

Stress reduction and moderate exercise are also important components of management.

Surgery is not recommended, and once controlled Crohn's can be managed long-term with moderately good success.

Colorectal Cancer

More commonly called colon or bowel cancer, colorectal cancer occurs in the presence of an uncontrolled mass of cell growth in the colon, rectum, or appendix.

The most obvious signs are rectal bleeding and anemia with marked changes in bowel habits and weight loss. The disease starts in the lining of the bowel, but if not detected, can spread through the muscle layers and then through the bowel wall.

Colonoscopy or sigmoidoscopy is recommended as a screening mechanism from ages 50-75. If the disease is confined within the colon wall, it is curable with surgery.

If the cancer has spread, however, treatment focuses on life extension with chemotherapy and other measures to enhance quality of life.

Colorectal cancer is the third most-diagnosed cancer in the world. Sixty percent of cases, however, are found in the developed world.

Irritable Bowel Syndrome

Also known as IBS or spastic colon, Irritable Bowel Syndrome is arrived at via an examination of existing symptoms and after excluding other conditions.

The syndrome is characterized by chronic abdominal pain and bloating and marked alteration of bowel habits which may include alternating episodes of diarrhea and constipation.

There is no cure, and treatment is based solely on symptom relief with dietary adjustments and psychological assistance as major components of management. Stress reduction is often critical to see real improvement in cases of IBS.

Celiac Disease

In people who are genetically disposed to suffer from the condition, Celiac Disease is an autoimmune disorder of the small intestine. It can occur at any time in life from middle infancy into old age.

The most obvious symptoms are digestive pain and discomfort marked by chronic constipation and diarrhea.

Children with Celiac will fail to thrive, and almost all patients will, at some time, exhibit anemia and extreme fatigue. Vitamin deficiencies are common, because the small intestine is unable to properly absorb nutrients.

The condition is caused by an allergic reaction to gluten protein, which must be completely removed from the diet for the patient to exhibit real recovery. Celiac is thought to affect about 1 in 1,750 people worldwide, but in the United States it is seen in 1 out of 105.

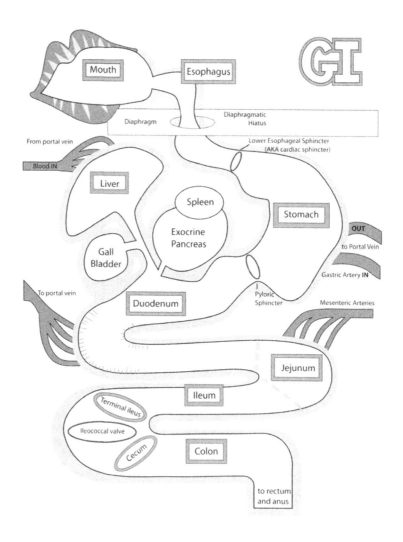

A rare bacterial infection, Whipple's attacks the gastrointestinal system and hampers its ability to absorb fats, carbohydrates, and other nutrients.

If left untreated with a course of antibiotics, Whipple's can spread to the brain, heart, eyes, and joints. In severe cases, the condition is fatal.

Symptoms include, but are not limited to abdominal pain and cramping (especially after meals), with diarrhea and accompanying weight loss.

The joints of the ankles, knees, and wrists may be inflamed. The patient will likely suffer from anemia with concurrent fatigue and weakness.

Little is known about the bacteria that causes Whipple's. It is seen most commonly in Caucasian men between the ages of 40 to 60 living in North America.

Gastrointestinal Defense Mechanisms

The human gastrointestinal system has many self-defense mechanisms. The highly acidic environment of the stomach is one of the most powerful of these, efficiently destroying any viable microbes before they have an opportunity to enter the small intestine.

Pancreatic enzymes, bile, and other intestinal secretions are also beneficial in killing unwanted microbes. The major assumption is that a healthy bowel will take care of removing any other potentially harmful bacteria or toxic agents.

The adherents of colonic cleansing believe, however, that the bowel needs help to accomplish this crucial task. That is where the concept of "autointoxication" comes into play.

The Theory of Autointoxification

Why does the bowel need help with cleansing? Because the modern diet is an exercise in self-poison. From fast foods and sodas to hidden pesticides, genetically modified organisms, and a veritable epidemic of gluten, the colon can't keep up.

In some discussions of the efficacy of colonic treatment, the bowel is likened to a sewer in danger of clogging up if the debris is not removed. If the "pipe" does back up, poisons literally sit in the body and pollute everything with which they come into contact.

The symptoms of autointoxication include:

- Food allergies and marked intolerance to others, including gluten.

- Frequent congestion.

- Flatulence or "wind."

- Low energy and fatigue that cannot be traced to any specific source.

- A weakened resistance to low-grade infections.

- Excessive sleep needs.

- Severe premenstrual syndrome and difficulty with menopause.

- Skin problems including acne.

While many of these same conditions can be caused by a myriad of other problems, they are often idiopathic — they appear out of the blue and no doctor can seem to find the exact reason way.

Why Consider Colonic Cleansing?

If you are one of the people suffering from an inexplicable illness, or if you are simply interested in preventing inflammation and disease in your body with a proactive program of alternative health care, there are many reasons to consider colonic cleansing.

- The procedure is universally promoted as a means of reducing stress. No one is happy when their digestion is functioning improperly. This can set up a vicious cycle. The more upset you get about your bad digestion, the worse your system functions.

- Colonics relieve constipation, which not only leads to a more comfortable lifestyle, but can prevent other, associated and uncomfortable conditions like hemorrhoids.

- Colonic cleansing has been found to improve the symptoms associated with a number of common digestive ailments including, but not limited so, Irritable Bowel Syndrome and Crohn's disease.

- The procedure will also remove parasites, which can often be a problem for people who travel through or work in underdeveloped regions of the world.

- Colonic hydrotherapy accomplishes an overall detoxification of the system by preventing the accumulation and buildup of poison in the bowel, which can then be seen into other parts of the body.

Other benefits anecdotally reported with colonic cleansing include improvements in conditions as wide ranging as bad breath to back pain.

The procedure can immediately erase the ill effects of taking a course of antibiotics, and relieve uncomfortable bloating.

Far from being a primitive bit of "quackery," the modern use of colonic cleansing via hydrotherapy and other methods including home treatment is a sophisticated approach to a problem that has been recognized for centuries.

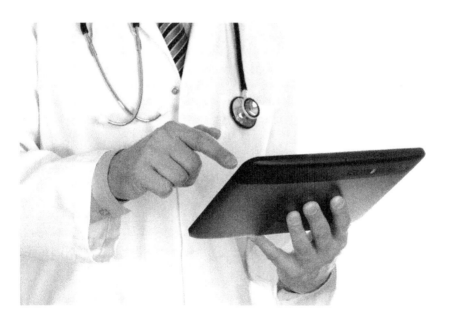

Mainstream medicine typically prescribes colon cleansing in preparation for medical procedures like a colonoscopy, but does not embrace the use of the therapy to detoxify the system.

The reasoning underlying this position is simple. The digestive system doesn't need any help to do what it's designed to do -- remove waste and bacteria.

Citing little concrete evidence to support the claimed benefits of colonic irrigation, doctors do point to potential harmful effects, including, but not limited to:

- abdominal cramping
- bloating
- nausea and vomiting
- a higher risk of dehydration
- electrolyte imbalances
- the potential for infection
- the danger of bowel perforations

For those patients that do elect to seek colonic hydrotherapy doctors offer the following cautions:

- Ask your physician if you are taking any medication whose affects would be altered by having colonic irrigation.

- Verify that the equipment that will be used for your colonic is disposable and has not been previously used with other clients.

- Find out if there are any herbal ingredients in the colon cleansing products to be used and investigate potential interactions with medications.

Above all, stay well hydrated prior to, during, and after the colonic. Since most people live in a state of mild dehydration on a daily basis, consuming plenty of fluids is good advice -- and good for general colon health -- any time, not just for the procedure itself.

It is impossible to over-emphasize the importance of hydration to good bowel function. Water constitutes more than 70% of human blood, muscle, fat, and bone mass.

We lose water through sweat and urination, and must constantly replenish our supply — a need most humans do not adequately meet.

The recommended minimum daily intake of water for an adult to properly digest food is

- 91 ounces for women (2.7 liters)
- 125 ounces for men (3.7 liters)

Most experts agree that it's best to try for 3 liters or 8-12 cups per day.

Losing as little as 2% of the water in our systems in relation to our body weight will decrease the volume of blood in our circulatory system and lead to constipation.

Drinking more water lubricates the intestines and softens fecal material for more efficient bowel response.

It usually takes around four to ten hours for your large intestine to absorb enough water from waste material, it is only then that can this can be to turned into partially solid stools. These partially solid stools consist mainly of water, mucous, fiber, and old cells from your intestinal lining. You need the water to flush this out, along with the millions of microorganisms present in your system.

Chapter 2 – Types of Colonic Irrigation

Studies in the United Kingdom have linked chronic constipation and associated digestive disorders to more than 300 conditions ranging from heart disease and cancer to arthritis and depression.

For years, naturopathic doctors pointed to the obvious anecdotal evidence of a connection between poor bowel health and broader systemic disorders.

Conventional medicine, however, was slow to accept the theory that accumulated toxins in the bowel could leak into the bloodstream, poisoning the body and touching off an autoimmune reaction.

Now, however, this idea, dubbed Leaky Gut Syndrome, is recognized as a contributing factor in a broad spectrum of physical and function diseases.

Even though leaky gut is still not taught as a diagnosis in medical school, practicing doctors are being forced to come around to the idea that rather than wage war on the body with powerful drugs that only aggravate the problem, the real point of focus should be on a good diet and healthy digestive function.

In an article by Matt McMillen, "Leaky Gut Syndrome: What Is It?" for the online medical reference site WebMD, Linda A. Lee, MD, a gastroenterologist and director of the

Johns Hopkins Integrative Medicine and Digestive Center said, " We don't know a lot but we know that [leaky gut] exists. In the absence of evidence, we don't know what it means or what therapies can directly address it."

In the same article, another gastroenterologist, Dr. Donald Kirby, director of the Center for Human Nutrition at the Cleveland Clinic said, "From an MD's standpoint, it's a very gray area. Physicians don't know enough about the gut, which is our biggest immune organ."

Such statements are maddening to practitioners of alternative medicine including colonic hydrotherapy, who do know what therapy will directly address and reverse the often devastating effects of leaky gut.

Leaky Gut Syndrome

Leaky Gut Syndrome affects the lining of the intestines, which is the first line of defense in the human immune system. The individual epithelial cells that form the outer layer of the intestinal lining are connected by structures called "tight junctures."

The microvilli at the tips of these cells absorb digested nutrients and carry them through the epithelial cells and into the bloodstream where they nourish the body.

In a digestive system that is functioning normally, the tight junctures remain closed and essentially screen the

---

molecules by only allowing them to pass into the bloodstream through the mucosa cells.

If, however, the tight junctures get stuck in an "open" position, the intestinal lining becomes too porous and cannot perform this filtering process. This allows bacteria, toxins, and partially digested fats and proteins to leak into the bloodstream. When that happens, the body's autoimmune reaction is triggered.

Autoimmune Response to Leaky Gut

As the gut begins to leak, the liver starts to work overtime in an effort to take up the slack and screen out the particles coming out of the intestine.

Unfortunately, the flow of waste is more than the liver can handle, and the undigested food, yeast, toxins, and other pathogens begin to accumulate in the body.

Although the immune system continues to wage war on the invaders, tissues throughout the body begin to absorb the material. Once that happens, widespread inflammation develops over time, stressing the system even more.

The Consequences of Leaky Gut

The longer the gut leaks, the more symptoms the individual experiences. These will likely include gas and bloating, chronic fatigue, joint pain, skin rashes, and growing sensitivity to foods.

Leaky gut can lead to Crohn's, celiac, rheumatoid arthritis, and asthma -- or make each of these conditions worse if they are already present. It has further been linked to:

- multiple sclerosis
- fibromyalgia
- autism
- chronic fatigue syndrome
- eczema
- dermatitis
- ulcerative colitis

If any form of inflammatory bowel disease is already present, the person is at a higher risk of developing leaky gut, which creates a vicious cycle of gastrointestinal issues. If food sensitivities to 8-12 items are present, you likely have leaky gut and don't even know it.

The Causes of Leaky Gut

The exact cause or causes of leaky gut are up for serious debate, but there do seem to be some common and known contributing factors.

Diet

High levels of refined sugars, processed foods packed with preservatives, refined flours, food dyes, and flavorings are all toxic agents that will increase the degree of inflammation and thus permeability in the digestive tract.

Stress

Ongoing stress is brutal on the body in a number of ways, and is especially hard on the digestive system. Stress leads to a suppression of the immune system, which means it cannot efficiently fight pathogens and is subject to being quickly overwhelmed and "outgunned."

Chronic Inflammation

Inflammation of any sort can lead to leaky gut. This irritation may be caused by low levels of stomach acid that lead to under-digested food passing into the small intestine to an overgrowth of yeast. Other culprits include bacterial, parasites, environmental toxins, and infection.

Yeast

Although yeast is a normally occurring flora in the gut, an overgrowth leads to the presence of multi-celled fungus that attaches to the intestinal lining and creates holes.

Zinc Deficiency

The intestinal lining requires zinc to remain strong. Without proper levels, the lining will weaken and become more subject to developing permeability.

Leaky gut may also result as a consequence of overuse of non-steroidal anti-inflammatory drugs, from the use of cytotoxic drugs, a course of radiation, certain antibiotics, and excessive consumption of alcohol.

Colonic Cleansing and Leaky Gut

Colonic hydrotherapy and the introduction of probiotics directly into the colon during the procedure are one of the most effective treatment combinations for healing the intestine and reversing leaky gut syndrome.

Colon cleansing encourages the bowel's natural function. Unlike an enema, hydrotherapy cleans the entire large intestine. As toxins are removed, the tight junctures begin to close again, removing the permeability and allowing for nutrients to be absorbed and filtered.

As the lining repairs itself, the action of peristalsis strengthens, and the colon begins to function normally again.

At the same time, all the corollary conditions caused by leaky gut begin to heal because the liver and immune system can now get ahead of the problem.

Rather than fighting a losing battle against a steady stream of toxins leaking from the intestine, the liver can cleanse the blood as it should, and the immune system can address and correct inflammation in the body.

Quick Facts - Antibiotics and Colon Function

The use of antibiotics can be extremely damaging to bowel function. Often antibiotics kill off the beneficial flora in the digestive tract. The human body should carry about 100 trillion of these helpful microorganisms in the intestines, however, according to a study published in 2012 by researchers at the Unversitat de Valencia, antibiotic treatment can irreversibly alter this symbiotic state.

Eleven days after antibiotic treatment is begun, gut flora reaches a minimum level after which it should then begin to re-establish itself. The research "shows for the first time, [however] that gut bacteria presents a lower capacity to produce proteins, as well as deficiencies in key activities, during and after the [antibiotic] treatment," researchers determined.

Although this study did not directly address the use of probiotics, this is a standard component of colonic hydrotherapy programs. According to the Harvard Family Health Guide:

"Probiotic therapy may also help people with Crohn's disease and irritable bowel syndrome. Clinical trial results are mixed, but several small studies suggest that certain probiotics may help maintain remission of ulcerative colitis and prevent relapse of Crohn's disease and the recurrence of pouchitis (a complication of surgery to treat ulcerative colitis). Because these disorders are so frustrating to treat, many people are giving probiotics a try before all the evidence is in for the particular strains they're using. More research is needed to find out which strains work best for what conditions." (*See "Health Benefits of Taking Probiotics at www.health.harvard.edu*)

Note: Since the health benefits are specific to the strain of probiotics used, it is best to consult with a qualified colonic health professional in selecting the probiotic best suited to assist with your particular digestive issue.

Particularly for individuals new to colonic therapy, deciding on the right approach can be both daunting and frightening. The most important thing is to locate a knowledgeable therapist you trust, but it's equally important to understand your options and what to expect from each therapeutic approach.

Closed Colonic System

In a closed-system colonic treatment, the client lies on a table very much like those used in massage therapy. The equipment used for the colonic is plumbed to an adjacent cabinet.

The therapist will insert a speculum, a metal or plastic instrument used to dilate the rectum. One end of a disposable hose is attached to the speculum and leads to the adjacent equipment.

Speculums are typically made of plastic and are also disposable. The average diameters employed for adult use are 0.60 to 0.65 inches (1.5 – 1.7 cm).

Some specialized sizes that are larger or smaller (for instance a 0.50 inch (1.27 cm) speculums for use with children) may still be manufactured of stainless steel and should always be sterilized in an autoclave unit after use.

The hose serves to deliver a pressurized stream of water into the colon. When the colon is filled, the water and waste material drains out of the body via the same hose and through an observation tube before entering the plumbing unit.

The therapist carefully monitors both the temperature of the water and the pressure level to guard against leaks and bowel perforations.

Although used with a wide variety of patients, the closed method is also preferred for patients who have suffered spinal injuries or who have lost full control of the anal sphincter muscles for any reason.

For patients suffering from constipation or a significant amount of gas, the closed method can be uncomfortable.

The majority of colonics administered in professional setting are conducted via the closed system.

Wood's Gravity Method

The most common of the closed systems is the Wood's Gravity method. It does not require the use of a machine, and is a more traditional approach to colonic irrigation. The treatment involves a tank (typically 5 gallons / 19 liter) tank suspended approximately 3 feet (0.9 meter) above the body.

Again, a speculum is inserted into the rectum, with a simultaneous in and out flow of water created that is controlled by the force of gravity only. The fecal material remains inside a closed tube and the patient is completely covered by a drape at all times.

The colonic is administered by a trained therapist who also applies abdominal massage as needed and/or pulsation of the tube to mimic the natural action of peristalsis in the bowel. This action is believed to tone and strengthen the colon.

Open Colonic System

Although there is some debate about the effectiveness of open systems because they do not cleanse as much of the bowel, this method does afford greater privacy for the client, and is generally regarded as more comfortable.

In an open colonic system, the client lies on a specially molded fiberglass table that resembles a recliner. The most common form of this treatment is the LIBBE system.

LIBBE System

In the LIBBE system the disposable rectal tube passes through a basin cut out in the chair. The tube is roughly the same width as a pencil. The therapist will instruct the client on the gentle insertion of the tube into the rectum before leaving the room to ensure privacy.

The therapist returns to the treatment room only when the client is ready, at which time a continuous gravity-fed flow of water is initiated through the tube. At the point at which the client feels a sense of fullness, they simply push to expel softened waste material.

The tube shifts to the side to allow the waste to flow into the basin. The feces pass through a small clear viewing tube, but because the system includes an exhaust outtake, odor is not a problem.

During the initial treatment, the therapist remains in the room to answer questions and to help the patient understand the procedure. For future treatments, however, the therapist does not have to be present, affording a much greater level of discretion and privacy.

Being Nervous is Natural

It is only natural to be nervous before receiving your first colonic irrigation treatment. By the same token, you will likely be embarrassed.

No matter how much assurance you receive in advance about the discreet nature of these treatments, your anxiety will still be present until you've seen for yourself the professional way therapists address the procedure.

Finding a therapist whose manner you like, and who will patiently answer all your questions in advance is absolutely crucial. The more relaxed you are with the therapist, the less tension you will hold in your body.

After the first treatment, the vast majority of patients say they worried excessively for no reason, and that colonic therapy is nothing like the horrible procedure they envisioned. Most report considerable feelings of energy and even euphoria. It is also common for clients to experience a burst of energy and an overall sense of enhanced wellbeing.

Do not proceed with a colonic until all of your questions have been answered. Give yourself plenty of time to prepare quietly for your first treatment, and don't schedule anything pressing for later in the day.

Once you are accustomed to receiving a colonic, you will feel little need to restrict your activities on the day of a session.

Your therapist should ask numerous questions about your lifestyle and eating habits, and may prescribe supportive care like a series of probiotic dosages to enhance digestive function.

Typically the initial course of therapy will last several weeks, after which you will only need to visit your therapist a few times a year.

Other Cleansing Methods

In general, advanced colonic therapy does not advocate a reliance on enemas and laxatives, but turns to these methods only as ancillary options.

Enemas

During enema treatments, water is introduced into the colon under the force of gravity. The waste material is released into the toilet.

Enema bags are inexpensive and can be found in most retail pharmacies. They are portable and suitable for home or travel use, but the necessity to lie on the floor or in a bathtub is awkward.

After the tip of the bag is removed, the patient must transfer to the toilet to expel the waste material. Loss of control during this relocation can lead to considerable mess.

An alternate approach is the enema board, which allows the user to lie down while affording water control via a container which can be positioned at varying heights. This option is less messy, but more expensive and less portable.

Repeated enema treatments can cause the end of the colon to become distended and weaken over time.

The result is that the patient becomes addicted to the enema process in order to accomplish elimination.

Laxatives

Laxatives are oral preparations that act as purgatives. Although laxatives can be highly effective for cleansing, over the long-term they tend to over-stimulate the colon and weaken the natural action of peristalsis.

There is documented medical proof of the addictive quality of laxatives if not used with caution. Additionally, this method has a dehydrating effect on the overall system as water is drawn from all parts of the body by the medication.

Quick Facts - What to Expect

In a gravity or open colonic, clients are ushered into a private consultation room and settled on a comfortable massage table.

The therapist will explain all aspects of the procedure, and clients remain draped at all times. Steps are taken to ensure both physical and psychological comfort. These may include calming lighting, soothing music, and warmed blankets.

Using a lubricated speculum, the therapist inserts two tubes into the rectum, one through which water will gently flow into the colon and the other for waste to be channeled into the drainage system.

An exhaust system prevents any unpleasant odor, and the therapist may administer abdominal message or gentle pulsation with the tube to stimulate the action of the bowel.

The consultations typically include counseling on diet and exercise, as well as instructions for after-colonic care. Most people do not experience any limitation in their normal activities after a treatment session. Most sessions last an hour or less.

In pressurized or closed colonics, the client reclines on a special chair into which a basin has been cut out. The therapist explains all aspects of the machinery and instructs the client on the self-insertion of a lubricated nozzle.

The therapist then leaves the room. The client will remove their lower garments only and inset the required nozzle. If this is a first-time session, the therapist will return and begin the flow of water.

On second and subsequent sessions, it's common for the client to speak remotely to the therapist who begins the flow without being in the room.

The water enters the body gently and builds pressure gradually until the client feels "full," which is the same physical sensation of needed to have a bowel movement. The material is naturally released and moves around the nozzle and down into the basin drain.

The process is odorless and painless and is repeated several times over a session lasting roughly 45 minutes. At the end of the session the patient removes the nozzle and cleans off with supplied personal items before getting dressed.

A colon cleansing procedure like colonic hydrotherapy will leave you feeling lighter. You may even drop a pound or so, but to really embrace colon cleansing as an aspect of weight loss, you have to think about the foods you are consuming in relation to their digestibility.

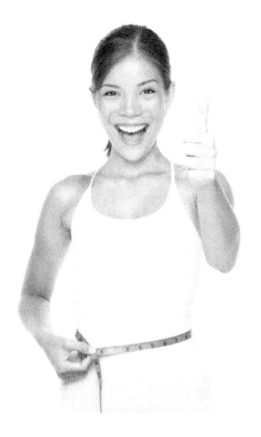

The modern diet is, for all practical purposes, comprised more of "food-like substances" than food. Every day we consume chemicals in the form of preservatives, dyes —

and even insecticides on vegetables that have been sprayed in the field.

Those same vegetables may well have been watered from a water table poisoned by pharmaceuticals and petrochemicals. At times, it can almost feel like a game of, "Which poison will hurt me the least?"

More and more health experts are extolling the benefits of a plant-based diet. Eating in that manner is the most naturally colon supportive and colon cleansing program possible, with the added advantage of normalizing your body weight!

A Colon Cleansing Diet

Colon cleansing diets are extremely healthy because they emphasize the consumption of greater amounts of high fiber. Certainly dietary fiber relieves constipation, but it is also instrumental in maintaining a healthy body weight while lowering your risk of developing both diabetes and heart disease. Additionally, finding satisfying foods that are also high in fiber is easy and not as restrictive as some eating programs.

Understanding Fiber

Also called "bulk" or "roughage," fiber is present in all plant-based foods. The body cannot digest or absorb fiber, so the material passes relatively intact through the colon and out of the body. There are two types of fiber:

- Soluble fiber can be dissolved in water. It is useful in lowering glucose and blood cholesterol. Dietary sources include oats, peas, apples, beans, citrus fruits, barley, carrots, and psyllium.

- Insoluble fiber increases the bulk of the stool in the colon and assists with movement in the bowel. Dietary sources include whole-wheat flour, wheat bran, beans, nuts, and vegetables like potatoes, cauliflower, and green beans.

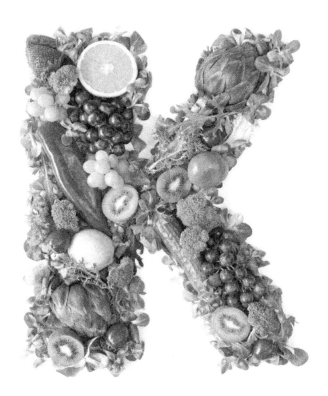

When you eat an item like beans or oatmeal, you're getting the benefit of both types of fiber. The greater variety of fiber present in the diet, the greater the benefits, which include:

- normal and regular bowel movements
- greater bowel health
- lower cholesterol levels
- controlled blood sugar

Although the research is not yet conclusive, high fiber content in the diet also seems to protect a person against colorectal cancer.

A high-fiber diet is excellent for maintaining a healthy weight! Fiber essentially gives your body time to get the message, "I'm full." Since most fiber-based foods require a fair amount of chewing, the brain can more effectively register satiety.

In 2012, the Institute of Medicine, a non-profit organization in the United States, recommended that men consume 38 grams of fiber daily up to age 50, and 30 grams a day for the remainder of life. Women need 25 grams of fiber a day to age 50, then 21 grams.

Goals of a Colon Cleansing Diet

When you concentrate on eating to protect your colon and promote weight loss, what you're really doing is waging a war on all the toxins present in the modern food supply.

Much of these materials come from a high concentration of processed items. (Smokers should work on quitting, and alcohol consumption should be limited or eliminated.)

Specific considerations with an eating program of this type include:

An avoidance of high-fat foods

Foods that are high in fat contribute to elevated blood pressure and weight gain, two critical factors in the eventual development of heart disease. Examples would include potato chips, French fries, anything slathered in butter, organ meats, and pork.

Processed foods

Items that have been canned or frozen not only contain chemicals and preservatives, but much of their nutritional value is lost. It is always better to eat a diet of fresh foods that contain no additives or so-called "stabilizers."

Caffeine

Caffeine is very detrimental to colon function because it has a constipating effect. Remember that caffeine doesn't just come from coffee, but can also be found in tea, soft drinks, and chocolate.

Sweets and candy

These items increase the body's production of insulin, which raises the risk of diabetes. Studies have found that about 76% of patients with diabetes also suffer from some form of gastrointestinal disorder.

Limit dairy products

Dairy products are hard to digest, even for those people who seem to "tolerate" the items well. Abstaining from or severely limiting dairy intake significantly reduces pressure on the digestive tract.

Above all, plan on drinking at least 8 full glasses of water a day. Good hydration is crucial for proper bowel function. Chronic, mild dehydration exists in near epidemic levels in the developed world thanks to the over-consumption of soda and coffee.

Specific Colon Cleanse Diets

It's no surprise that the diet section of your local bookstore is bulging with all kinds of books about eating for this or that goal. Colon cleansing is no exception. Often these plans are mixed with some form of juicing or detoxification.

Beware of any eating program that places long-term and intense demands on your total body systems. You must always consider, often in consultation with your doctor or health advisor, how any new diet will affect your total wellbeing.

Some books that will help you explore eating to cleanse the colon include, but are certainly not limited to:

- "Cleanse the Body: How to Cleanse with Body Cleansing and Colon Cleansing Juices" by Roy Silva

- "Detox Diet: Jump Start Your Weight Loss with This 7 Day Detox Diet and Guide to Detox Your Liver, Kidneys, Colon, and Skin" by Robert S. Mansfield

- "Eat to Live: The Amazing Nutrient-Rich Program for Fast and Sustained Weight Loss" by Joel Fuhrman

- "The Gerson Therapy: The Proven Nutritional Program for Cancer and Other Illnesses" by Charlotte Gerson

(For a short, 48-hour introduction to detoxing and colon cleansing, see "Dr. Oz's 48-Hour Weekend Cleanse at www.doctoroz.com/videos/48-hour-weekend-cleanse)

Good Colon Nutrition

By following the basic guidelines of good nutrition for the colon, weight loss will occur naturally over time. Studies have shown that slow and steady weight loss is more sustainable than rapid ups and downs on the scale.

Also, some substances, like gluten, that are irritating to the gut can take 6 months or longer to completely work their way out of you system.

Regardless of any diet "program" you might read about or choose to follow, the staples of sound colon health include:

Fruits and Vegetables

In addition to providing fiber, the nutrients in plant-based foods decrease inflammation in the body. They provide folate, which is a B-complex vitamin believed to decrease the risk of colon cancer, and they are high in antioxidants.

Whole Grains

Whole grain foods are high in fiber to assist with proper bowel function, and many "fortified" cereals also contain folate. Be careful, however. A high percentage of cereals are heavily sugared and processed. Make sure you're getting whole grains in healthy foods, not junk food by another name.

Fish

If you do eat meat, stay away from high-fat meats like pork, and red meats high in saturated fats. Opting for fish over these items will lower your risk of colorectal cancer while providing heart-healthy Omega-3.

The more natural, high-fiber foods in your diet the better. The effect of eating a primarily plant-based diet, with limited dairy and meats will not only trim your waistline, but it will greatly enhance the functioning of the bowel.

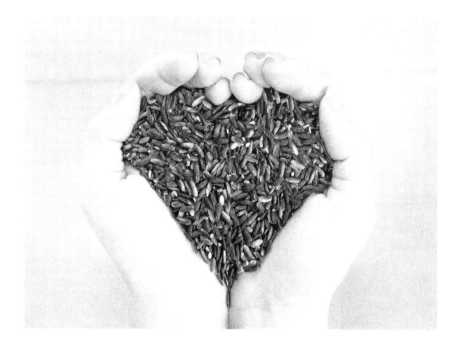

A healthy bowel not only allows you to extract necessary nutrients from the foods you eat, but it eliminates a prime source of inflammation — which is an open door to infections and autoimmune disease.

The weight loss aspect of a colon cleansing diet is certainly attractive, but the long-term health benefits are much more compelling!

The efficacy of colon irrigation and cleansing has been well established for centuries. The procedure should, however, be part of an overall approach to maintaining a healthy digestive system through diet and lifestyle.

The effect of healthy digestion on overall health cannot be over emphasized. With the prevalence of leaky gut syndrome in the developed world, and the unnatural condition of the modern diet, we are, essentially, poisoning ourselves with chemicals masquerading as food.

This, in turn, has created a near epidemic of autoimmune disorders that medical science often treats as inexplicable, rather than following the chain of evidence back to the body's first line of immune defense -- digestion.

In a medical culture that is prescription and procedure-based, the standard approach is reactive, not proactive. When "preventive" measures are advised, especially in regard to colon health, the philosophy is to recommend a method that is much more dangerous than colonic hydrotherapy -- the colonoscopy.

The Dangers of Colonoscopy

Colonoscopy is not the precise anti-cancer screening tool that medical advertising has made it out to be. It is, however, a $3000 /£1866 procedure, and thus highly profitable. Even in the face of well-documented evidence to the contrary, doctors still aggressively tout the "benefits" of colonoscopy rather than suggest the more effective, less invasive, and cheaper sigmoidoscopy costing $200/£125.

If their patients raise the issue of colon cleansing or hydrotherapy as a regular part of colon health? The same doctors who are praising a medical procedure that results in one death per 1,000 procedures will assure you that colon cleansing performed with nothing but purified, gentle irrigation is far and away the riskier option.

Where Polyps Are Located

Studies based on autopsy reports show that 35% of people eating a typical Western diet have colon polyps, two-thirds of which will located in the left or sigmoid colon and the rectum. Colonoscopy misses about 24% of polyps -- 12% of those will even be large polyps measuring 10 mm or more.

In 2009, the *Annals of Internal Medicine* published a study entitled, "Association of Colonoscopy and Death from Colorectal Cancer." The authors of the study determined that even though colonoscopy examines the entire length of the colon (five feet / 1.5 meters), instances in which cancer was prevented by polyp removal involved the last two feet / 0.6 meters of the colon.

A subsequent study, published in the *Lancet* in 2010, involved 170,432 participants between the ages of 55 and 64. Of those that received a sigmoidoscopy, a safer procedure performed with a flexible tube screening only the last portion of the colon, incidence of cancer was reduced 33% with a drop in mortality of 43%.

Colonoscopy as a follow-up procedure was used only with patients that met, among other criteria, polyps larger than 1 cm, three or more adenomas, and 20 or more hyper plastic polyps. Only 5.3% of the patients in the study required a colonoscopy.

The Real Cancer Risk

The risk of death to colorectal cancer is statistically less prevalent than the public had been led to believe. In 90% of cases, the cancers do not occur until age 55 or later. By that time, the growth has, on average, been transforming for 10-15 years.

Once it is cancerous, metastasis and death occurs in 10-20 years. The entire trajectory from normal cells, to cancer, to death requires 20-35 years. If one sigmoidoscopy is performed between age 55-64 and shows clear results, the individual will likely die of some other cause before colorectal cancer is a factor in their overall health.

Holistic Colon Care

Many of us fail to draw a conscious link between the emotions and colon health, even though we have all felt that instant nausea when we are scared or nervous. Many people don't like to get too far away from a bathroom when they're about to be faced with a big test or go in for an important interview.

This link between our emotions and our digestion can lead some people to make choices in the moment that have long-term effects on our health. When I was in school, the director of our speech department suffered from a very nervous bowel. In order to be able to attend and critique our performances for instructional purposes, she drank large amounts of over-the-counter anti-diarrhea medication.

While this decision quieted both her stomach and her nerves to achieve her short-term goals, over the long-term she developed chronic digestive issues relative to self-induced constipation that ultimately led to a diagnosis of bowel cancer.

In reality, my teacher was reacting much more to her panic over the prospect of being "sick." The "pink stuff" she was swallowing became a security blanket. The same can be said for people who eat antacids every day or who take medication for acid reflux disease. Some of the most common reasons people seek medical attention in the United States and the UK are:

- chronic bloating
- acid reflux
- constipation
- irritable bowel syndrome
- gastric ulcers

Each of these conditions is linked directly to a malfunctioning digestive tract, and each one increases a person's risk of developing leaky gut and subsequently an autoimmune disorder.

None of the recommended "treatments" will actually cure these problems, because they are symptom-based reactions, not proactive solutions for the underlying defect -- a colon that cannot work because it is inundated with toxins.

Proactive Colon Health

In addition to seeking colon cleansing therapy to remove accumulated toxins and strengthen the normal, healthy function of the bowel, consider all of the following measures to promote digestive health.

- Eat smaller meals on a more frequent basis: five times a day versus three.

- Drink as much water as you possibly can to keep toxins flushed out of your system. This will also keep your colon well hydrated, which is essential for proper function.

- Cut back on or eliminate alcohol altogether.

- Rather than using antacids or similar products, consider using a course of probiotics to re-establish normal bowel flora.

- Cut back on the amount of high glycemic index carbohydrates. These are foods that cause blood sugar levels to rise rapidly. Examples would be white breads and white rice, potatoes, parsnips, or anything containing glucose, maltose, and maltodextrins.

- Investigate your potential sensitivity to gluten by eliminating or greatly reducing your intact and monitoring how you feel.

- Increase your amount of dietary fiber derived from legumes, vegetables, and grains.

Investigate methods of stress reduction that will fit into your personal philosophy and lifestyle. This can range from a discipline like yoga or meditation, to taking a walk before a stressful event. What works for one person may not work for another, but it's important not to downplay the effect of your emotions and stress levels on your digestive health.

The Role of Exercise

Exercise, beyond its well established cardiovascular benefits, will also increase blood flow to your digestive tract. Additionally, that blood will be better oxygenated, better capable of carrying nutrients, and more resistant to toxins.

Walking, jogging, or running -- provided you have no existing joint problems -- are all highly recommended, but also consider sit ups and crunches. Over time, these abdominal exercises will give you the much desired "flat tummy," but more importantly, they strengthen your core muscles, which support the intestinal tract and enhance peristalic action.

All of these exercises can also help with chronic constipation. The more blood flowing to the area around the GI tract, the stronger the quality of the intestinal contractions needed for movement.

The Goal is Normal Function

One of the often cited concerns about colonic hydrotherapy is that the treatments become addictive: the patient can no longer function without the machine. Quite the opposite is true. The overall goal of a colon healthy lifestyle -- including the use of cleansing -- is to strengthen the bowel tract for normal function.

An initial course of colon cleansing, following by exercise, lifestyle, and emotional changes, will allow your GI tract to normalize so that over time, you will only need periodic cleanings for maintenance.

With clear evidence that bowel health is linked to overall wellbeing, the phrase "gut feeling" takes on new meaning. If your gut is feeling well, you will feel well. If your gut is filled with toxins, your overall health will be poisoned as well.

The real dangerous addiction is that created by the modern lifestyle -- chemical-laden, toxic filled food-like substances consumed at a breakneck pace under high stress conditions. This goes a long way toward explaining why so many people are overweight and suffering from "mystery" illnesses.

The third-century Essene gospel was right. *"The uncleanness within is greater than the uncleanness without."* To begin to heal yourself from the toxic effects of modern life, start with the place where the toxins have built up and are poisoning your system -- the colon.

Quick Facts: The Colon and Exercise

Failure to get adequate exercise will make the action of the bowel more sluggish. The more exercise you get on a regular basis, the less time it will take for food to move through the colon. This has a particular effect on the consistency of the stool. The longer it takes food to move through the system, the harder the stool will be and the greater the risk of constipation.

Do not exercise immediately after eating. Wait at least an hour. Immediately after a meal, the flow of blood to the stomach and intestines increases to aid in the digestive process. If you exercise, you'll divert that blood flow to the heart and muscles. This means:

- weaker muscles contractions in the gastrointestinal tract
- a diminished production of digestive enzymes
- sluggish movement of material in the intestines

Several conditions may results including:

- bloating
- gas
- constipation

Waiting to allow your food to digest, and then engaging in aerobic exercise will, however, enhance the function of your bowel. Simply walking 10-15 minutes 2-3 times a day will increase digestive function and colon health.

Other good aerobic exercises include:

- running / jogging
- swimming
- dancing
- aerobic machines (stair stepper, exercise bike, elliptical)

Yoga is a useful corollary to aerobic exercise aimed at good colon health as the gentle stretching tones the core and keeps the abdomen flexible.

Afterword

The "conveniences" of modern life have given colonic cleansing, a centuries old preventive health measure, new relevance in our lives. Food is no longer food, but a stew of chemicals and preservatives. Some are intended to extend shelf life, others are there by accident, the by-products of contaminated groundwater or the intentional use of insecticides on crops.

In the developed world, we are overweight and overloaded -- with toxins our systems cannot clean out on their own. The argument that, the human colon, by its natural design, is well equipped to do its jobs is true.

The entire digestive tract is a marvel of efficiency, from the point at which saliva begins to break down our meal for its journey down the esophagus to the stomach to the evacuation of useless waste.

In between lie the small and large intestine -- the colon -- and it is in those vital organs that so much can go wrong. The accumulation of poisonous debris in the bowel, called autointoxication, leads to a host of digestive diseases and conditions including leaky gut syndrome.

Leaky gut has been tied not just to autoimmune disease of all kinds, but even to attention deficit disorder (ADD) and autism. To neglect bowel health is to neglect overall health and wellbeing - the ramifications are that far reaching.

When performed by trained and licensed professionals, colonic hydrotherapy does not replace healthy bowel function -- it creates it. The procedure removes accumulated debris for the purpose of healing inflammation, closing leaky gut, and strengthening normal muscular action.

Over a period of treatments, when used in concert with corollary therapies like probiotics as well as diet and lifestyle changes, colonic hydrotherapy begins a process of reversal in the human system that can have staggering results.

Patients say they lose weight, sleep better, have decreased physical pains, improved skin, and even better mental function. Autoimmune diseases improve or resolve, and the system becomes highly resistant to disease.

Far from being a fad, colonic hydrotherapy in its modern form is an ancient therapy rediscovered. From the time of the Egyptians, regardless of the state of medical science, there has been an intuitive understanding of the role digestions plays in total health.

Detractors say the procedure is an unnecessary risk on one hand, while, on the other, promoting colonoscopy as a diagnostic method in spite to its overly invasive reach beyond the area of the bowel where most cancerous polyps are found. One in 1,000 colonoscopies ends in death, and 5 in 1,000 present with serious complications.

Colonic hydrotherapy is far less invasive, uses only the action of filtered water, and has proven long-term preventive health benefits with minimal risk. If there is no climate of inflammation in which a cancer can thrive, the danger is not just mitigated, it is removed.

It is an endemic flaw of modern medicine to react rather than to prevent, so colonic hydrotherapy seems to run counter to conventional "wisdom." In reality, it is a much older kind of wisdom, and one that has been proven -- literally for centuries -- to work.

Appendix 1 – Finding a Colonic Therapist

The following is a partial list. For a complete list of Colonic Hydrotherapists, please refer to The International Association for Colon Hydrotherapy at:

http://www.i-act.org

USA

Alabama

Stan Clements
STAN'S NATURALS
2305 Stemley Bridge Rd.
Pell City, AL 35128
Phone: 205-884-1160

Diane Deloris Brown R.N., MSN,
AQUA HEALING SOLUTIONS, INC.
1283 Circle St.
Dolomite, AL 35061
Phone: 205-744-7997

Diana Clark
MONTGOMERY COLON HYDROTHERAPY
7020 Sydney Curve
Montgomery, AL 36117
Phone: 334-264-6116

Renee Hughes
BODY LOGIC WELLNESS CENTER
5510 Hwy 280, ste. #202
Birmingham, AL 35242
Phone: 205-991-8083

Bernadine Suggs Birdsong
HEALING WATERS, INC.
720 23rd St., So
Bham, AL 35233
Phone: 205-323-7582

Queenie McNeil
A QUEEN'S TOUCH
1226 8th Street West
Birmingham, AL 35204
Phone: 205-323-9148 Fax: 205-323-9148

Ginger L. Bunn
BODY KNEADS THERAPEUTIC MASSAGE
209 Pelham Rd. South
Jacksonville, AL 36265
Phone: 256-782-2639 Fax: 256-782-2633

Neal F. Anderson
MONTGOMERY COLON HYDROTHERAPY
7020 Sydney Curve
Montgomery, AL 36117
Phone: 334-264-6116

Amelia Williams
HEALING WATERS, INC.
720 23rd Street South
Dolomite, AL 35233
Phone: 205-323-7582

Amanda Beth Mashburn
HOPE FOR LIFE, LLC
10300 Bailey Cove Rd., Ste. 7A
Huntsville, AL 35803
Phone: 256-270-8731

Linda K. Jarvis NMD
JARVIS NATURAL HEALTH CLINIC
1489 Slaughter Rd.
Madison, AL 35758
Phone: 256-837-3448 Fax: 256-837-3405

Deborah S. Taylor
OASIS SALON & SPA
891 Dykes Rd. South
Mobile, AL 36608
Phone: 251-607-9292

Alaska

Tina D. Williams
FEEL BETTER NATURALLY, LLC
1051 E. Bogard Rd., #14
Wasilla, AK 99654
Phone: 907-631-0530 Fax: 907-631-5200

Charlene A. Daniels
DREAM ACRES AK LLC
30630 Stubblefield Dr.
Soldotna, AK 99669
Phone: 907-598-4566

Kathleen Finn
WILD IRIS HEALTH CHOICES
1020 East End Rd.
Homer, AK 99603
Phone: 907-235-5329

Arkansas

Donna McElreath
NATURAL BODY INSTITUTE & ALLIANCE OF
CLASSICAL TEACHINGS
3115 JFK Blvd.
North Little Rock, AR 72116
Phone: 501-664-8200 Fax: 501-753-8202

Kimberly Sue Lowrey
GIBSON CHIROPRACTIC
93 W. Colt Square, #3
Fayetteville, AR 72703
Phone: 479-571-2656

Sharon Million
WHOLE BODY CLEANSE
2007 E. Nettleton
Jonesboro, AR 72401
Phone: 870-897-6070

Patricia Craig
NATURAL BODY INSTITUTE & ALLIANCE OF
CLASSICAL TEACHINGS
3115 J.F.K. Blvd.
North Little Rock, AR 72116
Phone: 501-664-8200 Fax: 501-664-8204

Joanne Bowles
MOJOME'S
3822 Hwy 7N, Suite 4
Hot Springs, AR 71909
Phone: 501-625-7458

Vickie L. Sims
BETTER HEALTH RESOURCES
312 N. Chestnut
Harrison, AR 72601
Phone: 870-365-3005

Arizona

Jacinda Jenene Aiken - MIND BODY & FLOW
290 South Alma School Rd., Ste. 11
Chandler , AZ 85224
Phone: 480-782-6566 Fax: 480-782-6463

Robin Bailey
NAMASTE SPA SEDONA
3080 Highway 89a
Sedona , AZ 86336
Phone: 928-554-4946

Alan Y. Murakami
THE BIODETOX CENTER
1000 W Apache Trail, Suite 121 (Thunderbird Plaza)
Apache Junction, AZ 85120
Phone: 480-288-9631

Jan Coleman
ALTERNATIVE WELLNESS CENTER
1400 N. Gilbert Rd., Ste. L
Gilbert, AZ 85234
Phone: 480-213-8374 Fax: 480-381-2222

Alice Ann Bachner
HYDRO-THERAPIES PLUS
1361 N. Lakeshore Dr.
Chandler, AZ 85226
Phone: 480-699-1917

Rose Lexa
ADVANCED COLON CARE & WELLNESS CENTER
2210 W. Southern Ave., Ste. A3
Mesa , AZ 85202
Phone: 480-844-0233

Teresa A. McConnell
ANTI-AGING THERAPIES OF AZ
1579 W. Lawrence Lane
Phoenix, AZ 85021
Phone: 623-451-0416

Rosalind Akins
ADVANCED COLON CARE
2210 W. Southern Ave., Ste. A-3
Mesa, AZ 85201
Phone: 480-844-0233

Benita Gettel
ECLECTIC BODY WORK
2127 E. Mabel St.
Tucson, AZ 85719
Phone: 520-795-6535

Aimee Reither
PHOENIX NATURAL MEDICINE & DETOX CENTER
301 W. Roosevelt Street, suite 2
Phoenix, AZ 85013
Phone: 602-307-0888 Fax: 602-307-1002

Maury Solomon
QUALITY MEDICAL SUPPLY, INC.
13372 W. Branff Lane
Surprise, AZ 85379
Phone: 623-640-4545

Dee Munsterman
COLON HYDROTHERAPY, LLC (LOCATED WITHIN
WELLSPRING HOLISTIC HEALTH)
430 W. Warner Rd., suite 104
Tempe, AZ 85284
Phone: 480-689-7744

Cassilda Tucker
1926 E. Velvet Dr.
Tempe, AZ 85284
Phone: 480-775-0595

Sheila Shea
INTESTINAL HEALTH INSTITUTE
4427 E. 5th St.
Tucson, AZ 85711
Phone: 520-325-9686

California

Angelene Fowler
THE HYDRATION STATION COLONICS
7708 Agate Beach Way
Antelope, CA 95843
Phone: 916-247-8859 Fax: 916-729-4220

Constance Jean Darlington
INFINITE HEALTH
20601 Hwy. 18, #137
Apple Valley, CA 92307
Phone: 310-857-8063

Pawnee D. Pleines
HEALING WATERS WELLNESS CENTERS INC.
2051 Hilltop Dr., Ste A11
2051 Hilltop Dr., Ste A11, CA 96002
Phone: 530-223-2322

Tammy Burt
VILLAGE MASSAGE
136 S. Halcyon Rd.
Arroyo Grande, CA 93420
Phone: 805-474-6082, 805-294-3140

Grace Lee
EAST & WEST MEDICAL CLINIC
30313 Canwood St., #23
Agoura Hills , CA 91301
Phone: 818-889-8988 Fax: 818-889-7787

Jamie E. Murphy
NATURALLY WELL
19063 US Hwy 18, ste. #105A
Apple Valley, CA 92307
Phone: 760-486-1976

Paula Schlue
BODYCENTRE
430 N. Lakeview Ave.
Anaheim, CA 92801
Phone: 714-974-1555 Fax: 714-974-9255

Tiffany Jablonski
NATURALLY WELL
19063 Hwy 18, suite 105A
Apple Valley, CA 92308
Phone: 760-221-5611

Edgar A. Guess, Jr. M.D., F.A.C.O.G
BEVERLY HILLS WELLNESS CENTER
328 S. Beverly Dr., Suite A
Beverly Hills, CA 90212
Phone: 310-284-8891

Veronica P. Wong
BEVERLY HILLS WELLNESS CENTER
328 S. Beverly Dr.
Beverly Hills, CA 90212
Phone: 310-284-8891

Mary (Molly) Leuthner
LOTUS ACUPUNCTURE AND HEALING ARTS
827 Bayside Rd.
Arcata, CA 95521
Phone: 707-672-3590

Maria del Carmen Sloan
KNEADED THERAPIES
31682 Railroad Canyon Rd., Ste. 6
Canyon Lake, CA 92587
Phone: 951-244-2528 Fax: 951-244-3981

Joy Day
BUKOVINA NATUROPATHIC MEDICINE
826 Lincoln Way
Auburn, CA 95603
Phone: 530-305-0897

Colorado

Anita R. Valenzuela
DISTINCT TOUCH
425 S. Sierra Madre St.
Colorado Springs, CO 80903
Phone: 719-471-3535

Madeline Angelus
ARTS FOR VIBRANT COLON HEALTH
2525 Arapahoe E4-621
Boulder, CO 80302
Phone: 303-243-4303

Melody B. Gibbs
PEACEFUL BALANCE
780 R Farmington Ave.
Farmington, CT 06032
Phone: 860-306-0051

Rebecca Richey RN
3770 S. Ulster St.
Denver, CO 80237
Phone: 303-507-6962

Julie L. House
119 E. Cooper Ave., Apt 30
Aspen, CO 81611-1762
Phone: 970-544-8054

Maureen Phifer
NATURAL HEALTH AND WELLNESS
7180 E. Orchard Road
Centennial, CO 80111
Phone: 303-221-2621 or 303-809-9754

James S. Allred
ADVANCED COLONIC TECHNIQUES SCHOOL AND
CLINIC
1750 30th Street, #35
Boulder, CO 80301
Phone: 303-325-6718

Todd Wagner
RETURNING BALANCE
2001 Blake St., Ste 2A
Glenwood Springs, CO 81601
Phone: 970-618-2492

Margaret Mazur
7855 Potomac Drive
Colorado Springs, CO 80920
Phone: 719-282-2330 Fax: 719-282-2330

Olivia R. Valenzuela ND
DISTINCT TOUCH
829 Sahwatch
Colorado Springs, CO 80903
Phone: 719-471-3535

Julie L. Roger
10177 Road 22.6
Cortez, CO 81321
Phone: 970-560-0160

Evelyn L. Gordon
THE SOURCE HEALING & SELF HELP CENTER
1761 Ogden St.
Denver, CO 80218
Phone: 303-863-9670 Fax: 303-863-8063

Connecticut

Bonnie M. Tetro
LONGEVITY WELLNESS THERAPIES
340 Scott Hill Rd.
Lebanon, CT 06249
Phone: 860-887-0215

Karen J. Laessig
ALAYA WELLNESS CENTER
535 East Putnam Ave.
Cos Cob, CT 06807
Phone: 203-992-1007

Patti Hartman
SHORELINE CENTER FOR WHOLELISTIC HEALTH
35 Boston St.
Guilford, CT 06437
Phone: 203-453-5520/203-500-0005 Fax: Ask about address at Wilton, CT

Constance Jones
GLASTONBURY NATUROPATHIC CENTER
18 School Street
Glastonbury, CT 06033
Phone: 860-287-4558

Jane Hefel
21 Lincoln Ave
Pawcatuck, CT 06379
Phone: 860-857-5022

Kelly M. Matthews
INTERNAL FOCUS WELLNESS CENTER
2913 Georgia Ave., NW
Washington, DC 20003
Phone: 202-234-7227

Dr. Hilda Perez
LOCATED AT ACHIEVE FITNESS/PERSONAL TRAINING
52 Waterbury Rd., Rt. 69
Prospect , CT 06712
Phone: 203-758-3470 or 203-241-4512

Michelle Sutton - Slatterey
THE COLONIC INSTITUTE OF WEST HARTFORD
43 North Main St.
West Hartford, CT 06107
Phone: 860-521-8831

Beverley Blass
JUST BE CENTER
12 Fairway
West Hartford, CT 06117
Phone: 860-206-1129

Ami C. Beach
COLONIC INSTITUTE OF WEST HARTFORD
43 North Main Street
West Hatford, CT 06107
Phone: 860-521-8831

Washington, DC

Sakiliba Mines M.D.
THE INSTITUTE OF MULTIDIMENSIONAL MEDICINE,
PLLC
2311 M. St., NW, Suite 202
Washington, DC 20037
Phone: 202-429-3783

Iya Makida Osae
NATIONAL INTEGRATED HEALTH ASSOCIATION
5225 Wisconsin Ave. NW, Ste. 402
Washington, DC 20015
Phone: 202-332-3100, 202-666-07690

Greta J. Fuller
WHITE ORCHID COLON HYDROTHERAPY, LLC
1352 Maple View Pl., S.E.
Washington, DC 20020
Phone: 202-669-6494 Fax: 202-889-3482

Kathy L. Vines
MEANINGFUL RELEASE WELLNESS CENTER
Washington, DC
Phone: 202-520-4934

Sandy Mitchell
NATURE'S RHYTHM, LLC
2111 Rhode Island Ave. NE
Washington, DC 20018
Phone: 202-635-2986

Sharon V. B. Roulhac
NATIONAL INTEGRATED HEALTH ASSOCIATES
5225 Wisconsin Ave. NW, Ste. 402
Washington, DC 20015
Phone: 202-237-7000

Martina C. Washington
NEW LIFE WELLNESS CENTER
426 8th St., SE 2nd Floor
Washington, DC 20003
Phone: 202-544-9595 Fax: 202-544-6820

Delaware

Cheryl L. Ciesa
25459 Draper Rd.
Milton, DE 19968
Phone: 302-329-9478 or 302-684-5423

Florida

Bernard Korn
AVENTURA NATURAL HEALTH & MASSAGE
20508 West Dixie Hwy.
Aventura, FL 33180
Phone: 305-466-0444

Candice A. Klein FL Lic #MA8163, MM4010
HEALTH CONNECTIONS MASSAGE & COLON
THERAPY
320 4th Avenue
Indialantic, FL 32903
Phone: 321-725-8347 Fax: 321-725-5191

Bonnie Barrett FL Lic# MA14802
RENEW LIFE
1153 NE Cleveland St.
Clearwater, FL 33755
Phone: 727-461-7227

Nancy Snyder
PARK AVENUE NATURAL DAY SPA
1401 Park Avenue, suite D
Fernandina Beach, FL 32034
Phone: 904-310-6788

Cathy Shea LMT, LCT, FL Lic. # MA12887
INTERNATIONAL SCHOOL OF COLON
HYDROTHERAPY, INC.
13878 Oleander Avenue
Juno Beach, FL 33408
Phone: 561-775-9912 Fax: 561-625-3775

Susan W. Herzfeld
FEEL THE HEAL
21300 West Dixie Hwy.
Aventura , FL 33180
Phone: 305-466-9268

Glenda Paulich
COLONICS WITH CARE, INC
8613 Old King Road South, Suite 302
Jacksonville, FL 32217
Phone: 904-739-9979

Norma Jean Barker FL Lic. # MA15155, MM 7322
NORMA JEAN BARKER, LMT, CT
5251 SE 113th Street
Belleview, FL 34420
Phone: 352-307-9720

Raymond Dotolo
DOTOLO RESEARCH CORPORATION
970 Harbor Lake Drive, Suite A
Safety Harbor, FL 34695
Phone: 800-237-8458 ext 2570/727-217-9200 Fax: 727-723-8888

Brian J. Lewis
INTEGRATED BODY WORK
322 South Marion Avenue
Lake City, FL 32025
Phone: 386-719-8887

Linda B. Griffith
REJUVENA
4501 Manatee Ave. W., #298
Bradenton, FL 34209
Phone: 706-455-3909

Rhonda Ford MA22058, MM9550
COCOA BEACH WELLNESS CENTER
236 N. Atlantic Ave.
Cocoa Beach, FL 32931-2963
Phone: 321-698-1519

Georgia

Karla Hoffman Magruder
BIONATURALLY
3645 Aubusson Trace
Johns Creek, GA 30022
Phone: 770-649-0789 Fax: 770-649-9119

April M. Hill
WATER OF LIFE, INC.
2510 Archwood Dr., Suite 12
Albany, GA 31707
Phone: 229-888-8272

Celia B. Lapovsky
PACES THERAPEUTIC CENTER
1 Galleria Pkwy- Ste #1-D7
Atlanta, GA 30339
Phone: 770-984-2332

Teresa Ducoffe
ATLANTIC COLONIC & MASSAGE
6710 Jamestown Dr.
Alpharetta, GA 30005
Phone: 770-558-6900

Mary Flory
AGAPE GARDENS COLON LAVAGE, LLC
Hampton, GA 30228
Phone: 770-228-2231

Maryann Wilson
WELLSPA SUITES
351 Thornton Road, suite 106
Lithia Springs, GA 30122
Phone: 770-948-8000 Fax: 770-948-9598

Candace Layer
ATLANTIC COLONIC & MASSAGE
6710 Jamestown Dr.
Alpharetta, GA 30005
Phone: 770-558-6900

Tasha M. Roberts
HADIYA WELLNESS, LLC
2048C Hosea L Williams Drive
Atlanta, GA 30317
Phone: 404-946-8552

Lawren Young
LAVIRI DETOX THERAPY
516 McDonough Rd.
Fayetteville, GA 30214
Phone: 770-316-2362

Pam Craig B.Sci.
ALLIANCE OF CLASSICAL TEACHINGS
285 Centennial Olympic Pk. Dr. NW, ste. #1807
Atlanta, GA 30313
Phone: 770-714-6350

Ilan Irie
HEALING WATERS INTERNAL FITNESS CENTER
Progressive Medical Group 4646 N. Shallowford Rd.
Atlanta , GA 30338
Phone: 770-676-6000

Meschell Perkins
YAHSHUA SPA & WELLNESS SALON
4500 Hugh Howell Rd., #320
Tucker , GA 30084
Phone: 678-226-3778 Fax: 678-669-1827

Hawaii

Shelley St. John R.N.
ST JOHN RADIANT HEALTH
P.O. Box 717
Haiku, HI 96708
Phone: 808-281-9156 Fax: 808-572-2463

Susan Gyan Bohannon
BAMBOO MOUNTAIN SANCTUARY
1111 Kaupakalua Rd.
Haiku, HI 96708
Phone: 808-268-2738

Alcyone Aquarian
HEALTH PROMOTION RESOURCE
204 Kuulei Rd.
Kailua, HI 96734
Phone: 808-261-4511

Cecilia B. Palos
BLISSFUL HEALTH, LLC
18-3821 South Kulani Road
Mountain View, HI 96771
Phone: 808-968-6755

Annalia Russell
A CENTER 4 WELL BEING
Kapa'a, HI 96746
Phone: 808-822-2686

Laurieanne H. Greig
NEW PHAZE (AT ALII MASSAGE)
75-5929 Alii Drive
Kailua Kona, HI 96745
Phone: 808-936-4999

Kaleinani Allen M.S., L.Ac., Dipl.Ac.
LANI'AINA WELLNESS CENTER
825 Kumulani Dr.
Kihei, HI 96753
Phone: 808-875-4669

Denise Janelle
TRINITY INNOVATIONS
PO Box 437298
Kamuela, HI 96743
Phone: 808-885-5699

Cindy F. Sellers
ANGEL FARMS
HCR 2 Box 6300
Keaau, HI 96749
Phone: 808-966-8581

JoDana P. Johnson
MAULI OLA WELLNESS CENTER
66-216 Sarrington Hwy, ste. #102
Waialua, HI 96791
Phone: 808-636-9004

Jo Kort
INTERNAL HEALING CENTER
Kapaa, HI
Phone: 808-823-9999

Anita Mitchell
NITAWELLNESSCOACH.COM
13-3775 Kalapana Hwy.
Pahoa, HI 96778
Phone: 808-937-2556

Mary Dressler
ALOHA AINA WELLNESS CENTER
P.O. Box 1720
Pahoa, HI 96778
Phone: 808-936-4555 Fax: 808-965-6696

Iowa

Teresa Baker RN, LMT
WELLNESS ESSENTIALS
2947 Four Seasons
Ft. Madison, IA 52627
Phone: 319-470-2305

Idaho

Kimberly George
LIVING WATERS
855 So Curtis
Boise, ID 83705
Phone: 208-378-9911

Juliana Plater Benner
HIGH STREAM HEALING
1617 N. 5th St.
Boise, ID 83702
Phone: 208-850-8075

Glenda F. Bell
LOTUS WELLNESS THERAPIES
2000 S. Longmont Ave.
Boise, ID 83706
Phone: 208-250-7670

Lorie D. Howard
VITAL HEALTH & WELLNESS CENTER
1865 East Sibley Blvd, Unit 1
Calumet City, IL 60409
Phone: 708-730-9040 Fax: 708-730-9041

Kimberly George
LIVING WATERS
855 So Curtis
Boise, ID 83705
Phone: 208-378-9911

Susann M. Clark
CLEARWATER COLONIC THERAPY
1639 Grelle Ave
Lewiston, ID 83501
Phone: 208-305-6705

Regina Danielsson
510 N. 4th Ave.
Sandpoint, ID 83864
Phone: 208-265-4194

Dr. Linda Mae Harms ND
DRUGLESS HEALTHCARE - COLON HYDROTHERAPY -
OPTICAL - MASTER BARBER
174 East Main
Wendell, ID 83355
Phone: 208-539-9563

Mary Farbo
SACRED FUSION, LLC
150 E. Aikens Road
Eagle, ID 83616
Phone: 208-941-1064

Cassandra Orjala
RADIANT HEALTH RETREAT
1291 S. Breezy Way
Post Falls, ID 83854
Phone: 208-640-4668

Opal L. Mortensen
ALTERNATIVE TIMES, LLC
676 Shoup Ave. West, Suite #14
Twin Falls, ID 83301
Phone: 208-733-6725

Illinois

Dorothy Chandler
PREP PARTNERS CONSULTING & TRAINING
11701 South Bell Ave.
Chicago, IL 60643
Phone: 312-238-9817 Fax: 877-366-8117

Steven J. Stryker M.D.
DIGESTIQUE
680 N. Lake Shore, Suite 1202
Chicago , IL 60611
Phone: 312-943-5427

Dr. Milton Chandler DN
PREP PARTNERS CONSULTING & TRAINING
11701 South Bell Ave.
Chicago, IL 60643
Phone: 312-238-9817 Fax: 877-366-8117

Starr Knight
KARYN'S
1901 N. Halstead
Chicago, IL 60641
Phone: 312-255-1590

Kimberly Randiev
CHICAGO INTERNAL CLEANSING
200 N. Michigan Ave., Ste. 404A
Chicago, IL 60601
Phone: 312-445-9569

Deborah A. Bamberg-House
WHOLE HEALTH NETWORK LLC
322 Burr Ridge Pkwy
Burr Ridge, IL 60527
Phone: 630-202-3603 or 630-307-3348 or 630-307-3349

Connie M. Lambert
CML WELLNESS CENTER
3925 75th St.
Aurora, IL 60504
Phone: 630-836-5257

Shelley Carlson
TOTAL HEALTH INSTITUTE
23 W. 525 St. Charles Rd.
Carol Stream, IL 60188
Phone: 630-871-0000

Nina Nicolai
INTEGRATED FITNESS -LINCOLN-PETERSON
MEDICAL BUILDING
5962 North Lincoln Ave., Ste. L-4
Chicago, IL 60659
Phone: 773-728-6800

THE MOVEMENT COLON HYGIENE CENTER
835 Virginia Rd., Ste. B
Crystal Lake, IL 60014
Phone: 815-679-0016

Jessica Eunhae Park
COLON CLINIC & WELLNESS CENTER
1430 W. Belmont
Chicago, IL 60657
Phone: 773-880-9640

Jodi Polo-Santiago
INTEGRATED CARE & WELLNESS CENTER
5011 N. Lincoln Ave
Chicago, IL 60625
Phone: 708-837-1800

Kansas

Laurie Black
YOU... ONLY BETTER
13622 W. 95th St.
Lenexa, KS 66215
Phone: 913-661-7147

Alice A. Herrin
NEW AGE HEALTH
9800 N. Halstead
Hutchinson, KS 67502
Phone: 620-543-6769

Angel D. Canady
NATURAL HIGH
9341 W. 75th Street
Overland Park, KS 66204
Phone: 913-901-8699

Caroline Cawrey - CAROLINE'S COLON HEALTH
CARE/YOUR WELLNESS CONNECTION
7410 Switzer St.
Shawnee, KS 66203
Phone: 913-422-8500

Angel D. Block
NATURAL HIGH
9341 W. 75th Street
Overland Park, KS 66204
Phone: 913-901-8699

Kentucky

Alison T. Szewczyk
BEREA HEALING ALTERNATIVES
111 Phillips St
Berea , KY 40403
Phone: 859-248-5739

Patty Biles
WORLD OF WELLNESS
433 Pine Ridge
Harold , KY 41635
Phone: 606-478-4745

Lillian Holliger
4010 Dupont Cir #5l8
Louisville, KY 40207
Phone: 502-893-2006 Fax: 502-893-9196

Karen L. Fessler
COLONICS OF NORTHERN KENTUCKY (VERY CLOSE
TO CINCINNATI, OH)
562-A Buttermilk Pike
Crescent Springs, KY 41017
Phone: 859-344-9997

Anna L. Roberts Hagewood
ROBERTS HEALTH FOODS
1020 Industry Rd., Ste. 10
Lexington, KY 40505
Phone: 859-253-0012 Fax: 859-253-1888

Louisiana

Sara G. Coleman
DESTINY DAY SPA
210 Plaza Loop
Bossier City, LA 71111
Phone: 318-752-2639 Fax: 318-752-2637

Randolph J. Bonvillain, Sr. LMT
LA PLACE HEALTH & BEAUTY, LLC
217 Melody Dr.
Houma, LA 70363
Phone: 985-872-0197

Carolyne Yakaboski
NATURAL WELLNESS CENTER
405 Stella St., Ste. C
West Monroe , LA 71241
Phone: 318-387-3000 Fax: 318-387-3030

Margie H. Ford
UTOPIAN COLON HYDROTHERAPY
15049 Florida Blvd.
Baton Rouge, LA 70819
Phone: 225-272-4447 Fax: 225-923-8704

Rose Williams
LE BON SANTE' WELLNESS CENTRE'
938 Chey Dr.
Lake Charles, LA 70611
Phone: 337-433-3330

Yoshida Moore
A NEW "U" WELLNESS CENTER AND SPA
1513 Line Ave., Ste. 334
Shreveport, LA 71101
Phone: 318-349-1926

Mary A. Williams
AZISA COLONIC DAY SPA
347 Acorn St.
Boutte, LA 70039
Phone: 985-785-2090

Marshall Meggs Sr.
HOLISTIC LIFE
4401 Veterans Blvd., #200
Metairie, LA 70006
Phone: 504-885-8800

Diane C. Kimbell
ALORACLEANSE
1131 S. Tyler St.
Covington, LA 70433
Phone: 985-809-3133 Fax: 985-778-0524

Brandon E. Bruce
DESTINY DAY SPA & SALON
210 Plaza Loop @ Louisiana Boardwalk
Bossier City, LA 71111
Phone: 318-752-2639 Fax: 318-752-2637

Kandyl K. Domangue BS, OTR/L
ALORACLEANSE
1131 S. Tyler St., Unit 10
Covington, LA 70433
Phone: 985-809-3133 Fax: 985-792-7186

Massachusetts

Valerie Jackson RN - NATURALLY CLEAN COLON CARE
CENTER (WHITE MARSH PROFESSIONAL CENTER)
7939 Honeygo Blvd., Building 3, ste. #223
Nottingham, MD 21236
Phone: 410-933-5858

Nancy Van Laarhoven
HEALTH WISE
165 County Rd
Lakeville , MA 02347
Phone: 508-947-1181

Marian Payant
BODY BASICS
945 Phillips Rd.
New Bedford, MA 02745
Phone: 508-985-9970

Pamela McDermott
CAPE COLON HYDROTHERAPY
East Sandwich, MA 02537

Romunda D. Ings
INTERNAL LIFE DETOX
9171 Central Ave., #L4
Capital Heights, MD 20743
Phone: 202-498-5339

Melanie D. Lewis
THE NATURAL PATH ALTERNATIVE, INC.
214 Market St.
Brighton, MA 02135
Phone: 617-787-5040 Fax: 617-787-5834

Lynn D. Munroe LPN
NEW LIFE SERVICES
696 Plain St., Suite 2A
Marshfield, MA 02050
Phone: 781-837-4316

Colleen A. Sackheim
STARLIGHT HEALING ARTS
20 Gore Ave.
Hatfield, MA 01038
Phone: 413-247-9689

Tami Johnson
INSIDE OUT HEALTH
12 West Grove St
Middleboro, MA 02346
Phone: 508-923-1030

Rebecca Ryan
BODY ESSENTIALS
25 Post Office Road
Chatham, MA 02633
Phone: 508-237-3302

Donna M. Behrle
NATURAL PATH ALTERNATIVES
214 Market St.
Brighton, MA 02135
Phone: 617-787-5040 Fax: 508-787-5834

Rebecca Martinez
THE NATURAL PATH ALTERNATIVE, INC.
214 Market St.
Brighton, MA 02135
Phone: 617-787-5040 Fax: 617-787-5834

Maryland

Nicole Gordon
NICOLE J GORDON HEALTH
10440 Shaker Dr., Ste. 105
Columbia, MD 21046
Phone: 973-271-7415

Tangene Sumlin
ST. JOHN ACADEMY
7711 Hillmeade Rd.
Bowie, MD 20720
Phone: 301-262-5303

Viviana Brown
ENOMIS OASIS WELLNESS SPA
6201 Greenbelt Rd., ste.#U7
College Park , MD 20740
Phone: 301-313-0012

Wendy Kurtz
WELL WITH WENDY
6302 Falls Rd. (within Sunlight Natural Health Center)
Baltimore, MD 21209
Phone: 410-277-1556

William S. Mussenden
ST JOHN'S COLONIC CENTER
7711 Hill Meade Rd.
Bowie, MD 20720
Phone: 301-262-5303

Petronilo A. Abiera D.C.
ST. JOHN'S
7711 Hillmeade Road
Bowie, MD 20720
Phone: 301-262-5303

Carl DeVonish
CLEANSING WATERS WELLNESS, LLC
2803 Eliston St.
Bowie, MD 20716
Phone: 240-375-7614

Sydney L. Vallentyne
ST JOHN'S COLONIC CENTER
7711 Hillmeade Rd.
Bowie, MD 20720
Phone: 301-262-5303

Mary Sczuka
THE HEALING PATH
1623 York Road
Timonium, MD 21093
Phone: 410-637-3760

Estrelita Stanfield
ANGEL HANDS
14 E. Pleasant Hill Rd.
Owings Mills, MD 21117
Phone: 443-642-0284, 410-599-2699

Pamela Reynolds
INSPIRED THRU NATURE, LLC
7301-A Hanover Parkway
Greenbelt, MD 20770
Phone: 301-345-1978

Valerie Kay Lancaster RN, CMT
HEALING SPIRIT HANDS
2795 Adelina Rd.
Prince Frederick, MD 20678
Phone: 410-535-0574

Chuck D. Anderson
SENSATIONAL TOUCH / HEALTHY WATERS
9636 Pennsylvania Ave.
Upper Marlboro, MD 20772
Phone: 301-599-0076

Maine

Elsie Cebulla
THOTHAN WATERS, LLC
PO Box 323
Shapleigh, ME 04076
Phone: 207-651-3171

Jody Ferreira D.C.
NATURAL CARE CHIROPRACTIC & ACCUPUNCTURE
6 Seeley Lane
Eliot, ME 03903
Phone: 207-439-9242

Michigan

Dawn A. Ford
STEPPING STONES TO HEALTH, LLC
7397 W. Blue Rd., Suite C
Lake City, MI 49651
Phone: 231-878-6601 Fax: 231-839-3210

A. J. Williams
MICHIGAN WHOLISTIC CENTER
1154 N. Ballinger Hwy.
Flint, MI 48504
Phone: 810-341-1902

Cheryl L. Cowsert
ECLIPSE FAMILY WELLNESS CENTER
125 S. State St.
Caro, MI 48723
Phone: 989-670-0814

Nancy Gurney
CREATIVE LIFEFLOW
280 Collingwood Dr.
Ann Arbor, MI 48103
Phone: 734-674-0922

Mary S. Echeverry Villa
MICHIGAN WHOLISTIC CENTER
1154 N. Ballenger
Flint, MI 48504
Phone: 810-750-6969 Fax: 810-341-1906

Brandy Boehmer
BIOENERGY MEDICAL CENTER
412 Longshore Dr.
Ann Arbor, MI 48105
Phone: 734-995-3200

Myroslava Bertalan
246 Bauman Ave.
Clawson, MI 48017-2004
Phone: 248-577-5889

Gil J. Bell
TOTAL HEALTH INTERNATIONAL, LLC
14547 Main St.
Buchanan, MI 49107
Phone: 269-695-3363 Fax: 269-695-3383

Ashima Rae
NEW WAVE LIVING
6563 Edgewater Dr.
Erie, MI 48133
Phone: 419-490-3870

Denise Whitman Elam
ENERGY 4 LIFE
16135 Mack Avenue
Detroit, MI 48224
Phone: 313-640-5790

Colleen K. Bell
TOTAL HEALTH INTERNATIONAL , LLC
14547 Main St.
Buchanan, MI 49107
Phone: 269-695-3363 Fax: 269-695-3383

Cheryl L. Cowsert
ECLIPSE FAMILY WELLNESS CENTER
125 S. State St.
Caro, MI 48723
Phone: 989-670-0814

Minnesota

Mary L. Montour
2142 Randolph Ave.
St. Paul, MN 55105
Phone: 651-698-3309

Renee L. Bergman
LIFE CLEANSE OF ANOKA
2665 4th Ave. N, Ste. 101
Anoka, MN 55303
Phone: 763-231-7303

Tammy Fischer
PEACEFUL WATERS WELLNESS SPA, LLC
7300 Hudson Blvd., Ste 220
Oakdale, MN 55128
Phone: 651-330-9583

Barbara J. Abeler
LIFECLEANSE OF ANOKA
2665 4th Ave. N., Ste. 101
Anoka, MN 55303
Phone: 763-231-7303

Robyn D. Roeber
THE BIRCHES CLINIC FOR COLON HYDROTHERAPY
1891 E. US Highway 2
Grand Rapids, MN 55744
Phone: 218-259-6416 or 218-999-5120

Kristin Burich
HEALING WITHIN WELLNESS CENTER
3200 N. Lexington Ave.
Shoreview , MN 55126
Phone: 651-490-3347

Missouri

Carrie Whitelaw
OCEAN CLINICS
2315 Dougherty Ferry Road, Suite 107
St. Louis, MO 63122
Phone: 314-966-7570 Fax: 314-966-7788

George (Rick) McLarty, Jr.
HEALTHY CONNECTIONS
5133 South Campbell, Ste 205
Springfield, MO 65810
Phone: 417-890-9700

Kristine Tow
HOLISTIC FITNESS
7501 Murdoch Ave.
Shrewsbury, MO 63119
Phone: 314-647-3999, 248-797-9925

Lisa A. Brown
HOPE PLACE, LLC
20776 CR 110
Tina, MO 64682
Phone: 660-745-3195

Char K. Haacke
THE MASTERS NATURAL ALTERNATIVES
201 Abbott Lane
Branson, MO 65616
Phone: 417-336-0807

Patricia Ann Gregory
GREGORY'S HEALTHY ALTERNATIVES
517 N. Taylor Avenue
St. Louis, MO 63108
Phone: 314-367-5553

Maureen L. Hays R.N.
HEAD TO TOE WELLNESS CENTER, LLC
6577 S. Crenshaw Rd
Ozark (Springfield), MO 65721
Phone: 417-724-2222 Fax: 417-725-0239

Maria B. Borja
HOLISTIC FITNESS
7501 Murdoch Ave.
Shrewsbury, MO 63119
Phone: 314-647-3999

Sharon N. Peterson
HOLISTIC FITNESS
7501 Murdoch Ave.
Shrewsbury, MO 63119
Phone: 314-647-3999

Karen Gelb - HOLISTIC FITNESS
7501 Murdoch Ave
St. Louis, MO 63119
Phone: 314-647-3999

Linda F. Stowe RN BSN LMT
ANOINTED ALTERRNATIVE HEALTH CARE
3175 W. Berkeley
Springfield, MO 65807
Phone: 417-881-6221

Mississippi

LaRhonda N. White - OPTIMUM HEALTH INSTITUTE
(FOUNDER DR. JOSEPH WHITE, M.D.)
6501 Dogwood View Parkway
Jackson, MS 39213
Phone: 601-366-7447 or 601-291-9933

Ronnie Ingley
LIVING WATER NATURAL HEALING & HEALTH
SOLUTIONS
55-98 Place Blvd., Ste. C
Hattiesburg, MS 39402
Phone: 601-579-8630

Montana

Peggy Kalaris-Small
AQUA SOOTHE
103 Ponderosa Lane, Suite A
Kalispell, MT 59901
Phone: 406-752-3390

Marlena C. Spray
1111 S. 4th St
Hamilton, MT 59840
Phone: 406-363-6180

Holli Gembala
AQUASOOTHE COLON HYDROTHERAPY
103 Ponderosa Lane, Suite A
Kalispell, MT 59911
Phone: 406-756-0247

North Carolina

SUNRISE COLON HYDROTHERAPY
7325 W. Friendly Ave., #A-1
Greensboro, NC 27410
Phone: 336-482-0270

Jennifer K. Woods
ADAWEHI INSTITUTE
93 Adawehi Lane
Columbus , NC 28722
Phone: 828-280-6331

Bonni Leone
HEALTHY HABITS WELLNESS CENTER
20700 N. Main St., suite 100
Cornelius, NC 28031
Phone: 704-895-7777

Geri Maloney Edwards
G. EDWARDS
PO Box 5124
Hickory, NC 28603
Phone: 828-324-0489, 828-270-9876

Neal Carver
5342 Nix Creek Rd.
Marion, NC 28752
Phone: 828-738-3369

Darlene Barnes
WELLNESS 2000
11801 Harris Pointe Dr.
Charlotte, NC 28269
Phone: 704-921-0079

Donna Randolph
HEALTHY CONNECTION, INC.
3302 S. New Hope Road
Gastonia, NC 28056
Phone: 704-823-1577

Gabrielle Rosina Lena Diamante
INTESTINAL FITNESS
6400 Falls of Neuse Rd., Suite 201
Raleigh, NC 27615
Phone: 919-872-2110

Karen A. Toledo
TOTAL WELLNESS AT ANGEL'S TOUCH
211 Duncan Hill Commerce Center
Hendersonville, NC 28792
Phone: 828-215-6565 Fax: 828-891-8897

Jennifer Turner
MAITRI COLON HYDROTHERAPY
802 Fairview Rd., suite 500
Asheville, NC 28803
Phone: 828-298-4054

Darlene J. Holloway
ALTERNATIVE HEALTH SCHOOL & CLINIC
919 Kildair Farm Rd
Cary , NC 27511
Phone: 919-380-0023 Fax: 919-380-0023

Catherine Gayle Simard
CHARLOTTE COLON HYDROTHERAPY
942 West Hill St.
Charlotte, NC 28208
Phone: 704-858-4803

North Dakota

Monica Beauchane
CLEANSE FACTOR
915 Washington Ave.
Northwood, ND 58267
Phone: 218-779-3492

Nebraska

Janet Patterson-Schaub RN
NORTHEAST INTEGRATIVE MEDICINE (INNER
HARMONY COLON HYDROTHERAPY, LLC)
72 South River Road, Suite 102
Bedford, NH 03110
Phone: 603-647-0600 Fax: 603-647-0633

Linda Mokos LMT
ESSENTIAL BODY THERAPIES
2030 N. 72nd St.
Omaha, NE 68134
Phone: 402-933-6220

New Hampshire

Deborah J. Clark
COLONIC CONNECTION, LLC
127 Concord St. (Rt 202)
Peterborough, NH 03458
Phone: 603-924-4449 Fax: 603-924-4449

James Pope, Jr.
1683 NHRT 175
Thornton, NH 03285
Phone: 603-238-6623

Donna R. Liolis
ALTERNATIVES FOR LIFE CLINIC & DAY SPA
179 Webster Ave.
West Franklin, NH 03235
Phone: 603-934-4810

Diane Wright
FULL CIRCLE COLON HYDROTHERAPY
89 State Route 101A
Amherst, NH 03031
Phone: 603-672-2350

New Jersey

Carylann Bautz
ALLERGY & HEALTH SOLUTIONS
278 Tuckerton Rd.
Medford, NJ 08055
Phone: 609-654-4858

Irina Openchenko
VALDI SPA
26 Bloomfield Ave.
Denville, NJ 07834
Phone: 973-664-1441

Iesha M. Clinton
IRVINGTON FAMILY PRACTICE
8-12 Krotik Place
Irvington, NJ 07111
Phone: 973-373-3000 Fax: 973-399-8880

Valentina Van Poucke
VALDI SPA & TANNING SALON
26 Bloomfield Ave. suite 1
Denville, NJ 07834
Phone: 347-803-8067 Fax: 973-664-0680

Christine Daniero
INTERNAL HARMONY WELLNESS CENTER
1916 Rt. 70 East, Ste. 5
Cherry Hill, NJ 08003
Phone: 856-424-7774

Diane Bleimann RN, MSW
525 East Rt. 70, Ste 3-F - Brick Office Park
Brick, NJ 08732
Phone: 732-918-2199

Linda A. Uveges-Durren
A TOUCH OF WARMTH - HEALTY HARMONY
BALANCE CENTER
328 Amboy Ave., Suite B
Metuchen, NJ 08840
Phone: 732-429-0613

Mariana Cuello
NATURAL CARE HOLISTIC CENTER
128 Baldwin Ave., #1
Jersey City, NJ 07306
Phone: 201-702-9799

Helene Therese Diab
AMERICAN HOLISTIC HEALTH CARE
131 Millburn Ave.
Millburn, NJ 07041
Phone: 908-656-5827

Shaista Tahir
WELLNESS CONNECTION
26-07 Broadway, Suite 12
Fairlawn, NJ 07410
Phone: 201-982-4141

Sharda Sharma M.D.
SHARMA HOLISTIC MEDICAL CENTER
131 Millburn Ave.
Millburn, NJ 07041
Phone: 973-376-4500

Masoud Rastegar
NATURAL HEALTH SOLUTIONS, LLC.
1870 Route 70 E
Cherry Hill, NJ 08003
Phone: 856-489-5174

New Mexico

Celia Green
CIRCLE OF LIFE
912 Baca St.
Sante Fe, NM 87505
Phone: 505-986-0775

Kukana Yarnevich
KUKANA
8920 Matthew Ave., NE
Albuquerque, NM 87112
Phone: 505-298-1983

Heather D. Gant
LIFE VESSEL SANTA FE
66 Avenida Aldea
Santa Fe, NM 87507
Phone: 505-473-1200 Fax: 505-473-1676

Donna Chambers
BACK TO THE BASICS
1603 Main Street SW, ste. A
Los Lunas , NM 87031
Phone: 505-869-3901

Jo Scott-Arbuckle
CALMING WAY COLONICS AT NOBLE SPA
1211 10th St., #4
Alamogordo, NM 88310
Phone: 575-437-5175 or 575-415-7540

Annabel Maria Munoz
SANTA TERESA NATURAL COLON CENTER
P.O. Box 776
Santa Teresa, NM 88008
Phone: 505-589-3130

Janetta L. Pederson
ALPHA CENTER
715 E. Idaho, Bldg 3-C
Las Cruces, NM 88005

Freida Payne
HEALTHY CHOICES
205 W. Church St.
Carlsbad, NM 88220
Phone: 505-887-3291

Lenka Svec
360 MEDICINE
66 Avenida Aldea
Santa Fe, NM 87507
Phone: 505-795-7111 Fax: 505-795-7112

Jeanette Joyce
RIO CLEANSING THERAPY, LLC
4944 Night Hawk Court N.E.
Rio Rancho , NM 87144
Phone: 505-228-6625

Nevada

Dr. Rob Toledo
HENDERSON WELLNESS INC.
9895 S. Maryland Pkwy.
Las Vegas, NV 89183
Phone: 702-474-7400 Fax: 702-920-8465

Anna Williams
BODY BALANCE WELLNESS CENTER
1680 W. Williams
Fallon, NV 89406
Phone: 775-423-1122

Donna DeCarolis
LAS VEGAS COLON HYDROTHERAPY SCHOOL AND
CLINIC
1815 W. Charleston Blvd., Suite #5
Las Vegas, NV 89102
Phone: 702-471-0088 or 702-568-0088 Fax: 702-471-6451

Dell Williams
BODY BALANCE WELLNESS CENTER
1680 W. Williams
Fallon, NV 89406
Phone: 775-423-1122

Claudia A. Calzadilla
LAS VEGAS COLON HYDROTHERAPY SCHOOL AND
CLINIC
1815 W. Charleston Blvd., #5
Las Vegas, NV 89102
Phone: 702-471-0088

New York

Trisha Rossi N.D.
THE NATURAL ALTERNATIVE CENTER, INC.
310 West 72nd Street, Dr. Office Entrance
New York, NY 10023
Phone: 212-580-3333 Fax: 212-873-5891

Maria Goldenberg
NATURAL HEALTH & NUTRITION CENTER
2701 Ocean Ave.
Brooklyn , NY 11229
Phone: 718-336-2818 Fax: 718-336-2818

Larissa Sarjinskaia
NY
Phone: 718-864-9884

Cindy Jackson Van Valen
CINDY JACKSON VAN-VALEN
2280 Western Ave.
Guilderland, NY 12084
Phone: 518-456-4008

Ivan P. Eusebe
CIRCLE OF LIFE
711 Bristol St.
Brooklyn, NY 11236
Phone: 718-498-4024

Hilda Pichardo ND
MY WELLNESS SOLUTIONS
3044 Third Ave.
Bronx, NY 10451
Phone: 718-992-7741

Estrella Caban
INTEGRATIVE HEALING CENTER
1180 Northern Blvd.
Manhasset, NY 11030
Phone: 516-967-3142

Nancy Miller
400 Rugby Rd., #6-D
Brooklyn , NY 11226
Phone: 917-498-3591

Jaime Clifford
OPTIMAL WELLNESS CENTER
70 Glenn St. Ste. 240
Glen Cove, NY 11542
Phone: 516-801-4971

Elisa Street
MYTHS
26 W. Main St.
Middletown, NY 10940
Phone: 845-204-0377 Fax: 845-343-1897

Mary Sue Nahmias
NAHMIAS HEALTH AND WELLNESS, LLC
9 Paddock Dr.
Fort Salonga, NY 11768
Phone: 631-707-6402 Fax: 631-292-2463

Carol Drake
HEALTHY ENDINGS WELLNESS CENTER AND DAY
SPA
640 East 103rd St
Brooklyn, NY 11236
Phone: 718-272-8686

Alexandra Defacio
224 5th Avenue, 3rd Floor
New York, NY 10001
Phone: 212-213-8520, 917-476-4492

Ohio

Heasock Chung
GET WELL CENTER
635 S. Trimble Rd.
Mansfield, OH 44906
Phone: 419-524-2676

Nancy J. Block
STUBBENDIECK CHIROPRACTIC AND
REHABILITATION CENTERS
257 S. Court, Unit 5A
Medina , OH 44256
Phone: 330-725-4060

Trisha DeHall
CINCINNATI COLON HYDROTHERAPY
7923 Blue Ash Rd., suite A
Cincinnati, OH 45243
Phone: 513-356-6215 Fax: 513-297-9499

Vickie Lynn Gibbs
RADIANT LIVING
81 West Waterloo Street
Columbus, OH 43110
Phone: 740-654-3884

Linda J. Clifton-McCormick
"PRICELESS" HEALING HERBS
1611 Spring Valley Ave. NW
Canton, OH 44708
Phone: 330-477-6400

Lisa Gatto
SERENDIPITY QUALITY OF LIFE CENTER
1356 Eastview Ave. #B
Columbus, OH 43212
Phone: 614-288-9672

James Kendel DC, DABFP
MEDINA FAMILY CHIROPRACTIC CENTER
5019 Victor Dr.
Medina, OH 44256
Phone: 330-722-7709 Fax: 330-723-0850

Laura Ann Schaaf
PEACE AT HAND
502 E. Tiffin St., P.O. Box 362
Attica, OH 44807-0362
Phone: 567-224-1441

Connie Thrush
PEACE AT HAND
502 E. Tiffin St., P.O. Box 362
Attica, OH 44807-0362
Phone: 567-224-1441

Mary Clark
HOUSE OF REFLEXOLOGY AND MASSAGE THERAPY
7731 CR 29 East
Bellville, OH 44813
Phone: 419-362-8210

Robert C. Angus, Jr. B.Sc.
CELEBRATION OF HEALTH ASSN.
122 Thurman St.
Bluffton, OH 45817
Phone: 419-358-4627

Tamara R. Waller .
BACK TO BASICS
2420 2nd St. #3
Cuyahoga Falls, OH 44221
Phone: 330-608-8540

Oklahoma

Emile Spalitta
OASIS COLON HYDROTHERAPY
115 2nd St.
Talihina , OK 74571
Phone: 504-237-9699

Don Ed Little
BODY CONNECTION
322 1/2 N 3rd Ave
Durant, OK 74701
Phone: 580-745-9201

Joyce Alexander
BODY CONNECTION THERAPY
322 1/2 N. 3rd
Durant, OK 74701
Phone: 580-745-9201

Jamie Reed
FULL CIRCLE HEALTH
3601 S. Broadway #200
Edmond, OK 73013
Phone: 405-520-2929 Fax: 405-753-9478

Debbie Dise
COLON CARE CENTER OF OKLAHOMA
8316 E. 61st Street, Ste. 101
Tulsa, OK 74133
Phone: 918-872-8844, 918-207-5799 Fax: 918-872-8854

Terry M. Reed ND
BACK TO EDEN COUNSELING AND WELLNESS CTR
4605 N. MacArthur Blvd.
Warr Acres, OK 73122
Phone: 405-787-6111

Sigrid Myers
NATURCARE
1529 S. 112th E. Ave.
Tulsa, OK 74128
Phone: 918-437-3698

Oregon

Tara Lyn Alder
ALDER BROOKE HEALING ARTS
1477 Lake Dr.
Eugene , OR 97404
Phone: 541-513-7894

Rebecca Harder
COLON CARE, LLC
7105 SW Varns St., suite 100
Portland, OR 97223
Phone: 503-222-3311

Vicki Sorce
SORCE OF HEALTH COLON HYDROTHERAPY
832 E. Main St. Suite 7
Medford, OR 97504
Phone: 541-282-5828 Fax: 541-770-1327

Christy Garcia Santamaria
ALL'S WELL THAT ENDS WELL
316 NE 28th Ave.
Portland, OR 97217
Phone: 503-230-0812

Paddy Lazar
ALLS WELL THAT ENDS WELL
316 NE 28th Ave
Portland, OR 97232
Phone: 503-230-0812

Linda Marie McCullough
ESSENTIAL WATERS HEALING ARTS
1724 Lakeview Avenue
Klamath Falls, OR 97601
Phone: 541-273-0220 Fax: 541-273-0220

Kerie Raymond ND
HAWTHORN HEALING ARTS CENTER
39 NW Louisiana Ave
Bend, OR 97701
Phone: 541-504-0250 Fax: 541-330-6635

Cindy Kerbaugh
COLON CARE LLC
7105 SW Varns, suite 100
Portland , OR 97223
Phone: 360-703-1010

Sarah West
ASHLAND COLON HYDROTHERAPY CENTER
290 North Main Street, #7
Ashland, OR 97520
Phone: 541-201-0500

Maggie Marie Youngstrom-Lowry
SORCE OF HEALTH COLON HYDROTHERAPY
832 E. Main St., Ste. 7
Medford, OR 97504

Linda Frantz RN
AHIMSA BODY THERAPIES
155 NW Hawthorne Ave.
Bend, OR 97701
Phone: 541-610-5528

Marty Bigger
33314 S. E. Peoria Rd
Corvallis, OR 97333
Phone: 541-757-1454

Pennsylvania

Marlene D. Noullet
NOULLET'S HEALTH CENTER
227 Crisswell Road
Butler, PA 16001
Phone: 724-287-0687

Jenifer Cammauf
4 N. Conestoga View Drive
Akron, PA 17501
Phone: 717-859-1869

Sally J. Garber
13451 Sunrise Dr.
Blue Ridge Summit, PA 17214-9747
Phone: 717-794-2144

Arleen Patricia Ehritz
BEGIN WITHIN WELLNESS SPA
151 Hoffman Rd.
Barto, PA 19504
Phone: 610-754-1747

Linda K. Puder
THE D-STRESS STATION
111 Boal Ave.
Boalsburg, PA 16827
Phone: 814-466-1020

Karen Lea Brady
144 Bergad Lane Freeport
Freeport, PA 16229
Phone: 724-295-5591

Nancy E. Ardire
CLEANSING WATERS
2137 Orchard Rd.
Camp Hill, PA 17011
Phone: 717-926-0472

Sherry A. Wachter
PATHWAYS TRANSFORMATIONAL CENTER FOR
COLON HYDROTHERAPY
4833 Chestnut Street
Emmaus, PA 18049
Phone: 610-966-7001

Shelly Morasco
IN LIGHT STUDIO
170 Camp Stewart Road
Coatesville, PA 19320
Phone: 610-466-7733

Jamale Crockett
HEALTH ENHANCEMENT CO. LLC.
1341 West 26th St, Suite 200
Erie, PA 16508
Phone: 814-459-2030

Mary Anne Biehler
6500 Wissahickon Ave, #3 - L
Philadelphia, PA 19119
Phone: 215-843-4886

Susan P. Rubendall
CJ PATTON CENTER
15 Savidge Rd.
Millersburg, PA 17061
Phone: 717-362-2067 Fax: 717-362-3159

South Carolina

La Pointe La Pointe
INTERNATIONAL WELLNESS CLINIC
207 Brown Arrow Circle
Inman, SC 29349
Phone: 863-286-2204 Fax: 864-285-0902

Wendy Law
EASLEY THERAPEUTIC MASSAGE
P.O. Box 1334
Easley, SC 29640
Phone: 864-306-0336

Sally Thompson
PALMETTO WELLNESS
212 N. Logan
Gaffney, SC 29341
Phone: 864-489-9080

Jennifer Knowles
SYNERGY WELLNESS BOUTIQUE
101 Queen St., suite 100
Charleston, SC 29464
Phone: 843-345-7370

Thena M. Goode
AIKEN HYDROTHERAPY CENTER
380 Talatha Church Rd.
Aiken, SC 29803
Phone: 803-979-3574

Betsy S. Exton
COLON HYDRATION
14 South Main St.
Greenville, SC 29601
Phone: 864-233-4811

Brenda Gail Goode
AIKEN HYDROTHERAPY CENTER
380 A Talatha Church Rd.
Aiken, SC 29803
Phone: 803-641-6350 Fax: 803-641-6348

Helen Davis
GALLERY OF HEALTH
10 Enterprise Blvd., East Side Medical Center, ste. #207
Greenville, SC 29615
Phone: 864-232-0100

Sharon Fincke
A CENTER FOR WELL BEING
1830 Belgrade Avenue
Charleston, SC 29407
Phone: (843) 769-6848 Fax: (843) 762-6393

Melvin P. Jenkins, Jr.
INTERNAL CLEANSING AND HEALING CENTER
9400 Twonotch Rd., Ste. B
Columbia , SC 29223
Phone: 803-462-0707 Fax: 803-462-0709

Joan Geanuracos
A CENTER FOR WELL BEING
1830 Belgrade Avenue
Charleston, SC 29407
Phone: 843-769-6848

Phyllis P. Woods
INTERNAL FITNESS
400 S. Main St. Suite J
Maulden, SC 29662
Phone: 864-757-1269 or 864-386-1942

Dr. W. Claire Wages DC
BACK TO ESSENTIALS, LLC
Health and Wellness Center 1713 Taylor Street, Suite C
Columbia, SC 29201
Phone: 803-708-9674 Fax: 803-736-0923

Tennessee

Sharon Ruffin
TERIVIKHANDS
600 Pennsylvania Ave
Oak Ridge, TN 37830
Phone: 865-483-0121

Quinn Raines R.N.
WARM SPRINGS WELLNESS CENTER & SCHOOL
567 Cason Lane, Suite C-1
Murfreesboro, TN 37128
Phone: 615-426-0472

Anne Lee
TUMMY SOLUTIONS
225 E. Meadow Circle
Clarksville, TN 37043
Phone: 931-906-8083 Fax: 931-906-8284

Linda Roll-Smith
INNER HEALTH
1600 Bill Eller Dr.
LaVergne, TN 37086
Phone: 615-793-0134 / 615-336-6109

Celesta Ewin
HEALING AQUAS WELLNESS SOLUTIONS
1106 Ed Temple Blvd.
Nashville, TN 37208
Phone: 615-977-0613

Amber Sam Matthews
RENEW WELLNESS SPA
3040 Forest Hills Irene Rd., Ste. 109
Germantown, TN 38138
Phone: 901-435-6150

Linda Roll Smith
INNER HEALTH, LLC
1600 Bill Eller Dr.
LaVergne, TN 37086
Phone: 615-793-0134

Debbie Ritter
NEW LIFE PHYSICIANS
5055 Maryland Way
Brentwood, TN 37027
Phone: 615-771-8832 Fax: 615-771-7472

April Smalley
JOURNEY TO WELL BEING
213 Stecoah Court
Cane Ridge, TN 37013
Phone: 615-293-5063

Lorna Lewis
TUMMY SOLUTIONS
225 East Meadow Circle
Clarksville, TN 37043
Phone: 931-906-8083

Kathie Bauer
WHITE CREEK WELLNESS CENTER
332 Pine Flat Rd.
Deer Lodge, TN 37726
Phone: 423-965-4731 ext. 0 or 865-256-5113 Fax: 423-965-4731

Paula J. Perkins
1204 Frederick Dr.
Knoxville, TN 37931
Phone: 865-675-5530 or 865-951-9382

Texas

Donna J. Blue-Booker
MIND BODY CENTER & COLONIC NETWORK SCHOOL
(FORMERLY MIND BODY SCHOOL)
10911 West Ave
San Antonio, TX 78213
Phone: 210-308-8888

Roy Rocco Bruno
REGENESIS & LIFESTREAM COLON HYDROTHERAPY
INSTITUTE
2001 South Lamar, Ste G
Austin, TX 78704
Phone: 512-326-3737

Tracie Torres-Graves
NATURAL THERAPEUTICS
6340 Camp Bowie Blvd.
Fort Worth, TX 76116
Phone: 817-738-4904

Lillian Christian-Prothro
CHRISTIAN COLON CLEANING CENTRE
4702 Old Coach Lane
San Antonio, TX 78220
Phone: 210-661-2089

Garlyn E. Mayo
NATURAL THERAPEUTICS
6340 Camp Bowie Blvd.
Ft. Worth, TX 76116
Phone: 817-738-4904

Patricia K. Noble
ROCK SOLID HEALTH
1106 S Mays St, Ste.#210
Round Rock, TX 78664
Phone: 512-608-7325

Donna J. Otey
ALPHA CLEANSE
1302 W. Magnolia Ave.
Ft. Worth, TX 76104
Phone: 817-335-7700 Fax: 817-292-1392

Janice Jackson
INSIDE OUT & WITHIN
5515 Corporate Dr, Suite D1
Houston, TX 77036
Phone: 281-561-8181

Trena Ann Sims
NATURAL THERAPEUTICS
6340 Camp Bowie Blvd.
Fort Worth, TX 76116
Phone: 817-738-4904

Karen P. Million
LAKE TRAVIS WELLNESS CENTER
2903 Ranch Road 620 North
Austin, TX 78734
Phone: 512-266-9105

Charlotte A. Layne
3839 Bee Cave Rd., #202
Austin, TX 78746
Phone: 512-328-9849 Fax: 512-327-4944

Lynmarie Corbett
CHARLOTTE LAYNE
3839 Bee Cave Rd., Ste. 202
Austin, TX 78746
Phone: 512-810-0333

Utah

Carol Buma
1763 Quartz Dr.
St. George, UT 84790
Phone: 619-667-3600

Jill Whitley
LIGHTEN YOUR PATH
972 Chambers St., Suite 5
South Ogden, UT 84405
Phone: 801-458-3267

Danette Fry
LIGHTEN YOUR PATH
972 Chambers St., Suite 5
South Ogden, UT 84405
Phone: 801-458-3267

Uli Braun
INTERNAL BALANCE & UTAH SCHOOL OF COLON
HYDROTHERAPY
520 S. State St., Ste. M-4
Orem, UT 84058
Phone: 435-660-1180

Chad L. Hosler
INNERLIGHT
1364 W. 600 S.
Salt Lake City, UT 84104
Phone: 801-366-9544

Aubree J. Weeks
COLON HEALTH INSTITUTE
21 N. 490 West
American Fork, UT 84003
 USA
Phone: 801-822-1611

Judy Morgan
GENTLE COLON CARE
1659 North 900 West
West Bountiful (Salt Lake City Area), UT 84087
Phone: 801-295-9422

Karen M. Schiff PT
HEALTH WAVE
150 South. 600 East, Unit 1A
Salt Lake City, UT 84102
Phone: 801-541-3064

Mia Magistro
WHOLE BODY CLEANSING AND COLONICS
1103 South Orem Blvd.
Orem, UT 84058
Phone: 801-427-1049

Brigitte D. Aagard
HEALTH WAVE
150 S. 600 E., Suite 1A
Salt Lake City, UT 84102
Phone: 801-541-3064

Virginia

Susanne Hylen
MYLANDRE
208 N. Washington St.
Alexandria, VA 22314
Phone: 708-836-0679

Mylene Frances
ALEXANDRIA COLON CARE
208 N. Wasthington St.
Alexandria, VA 22314
Phone: 714-348-7719

Rebecca Danielle Wright
VITALITY CLEANSING, LLC.
44121 Harry Byrd Highway, #115
Ashburn, VA 20147

Caroline Elizabeth Alexander
VITALITY CLEANSING, LLC
44121 Harry Byrd. Highway, Suite 115
Ashburn, VA 20147
Phone: 571-331-1497

Felicia B. Asenso RN
HEALTH TALK, INC.
6130 Wicklow Dr.
Burke, VA 22015
Phone: 703-822-7471

Lorraine Pilarski
MANUAL MEDICAL THERAPIES
2418 Bay Oaks Place
Norfolk, VA 23518
Phone: 757-587-6062 Fax: 757-587-5306

Kathi Dawson Fentress
HELP FOR HEALTH
6116 Rolling Road, Suite 306B
Springfield, VA 22152
Phone: 703-644-4325 or 571-722-4971

Ariel C. Selwyn
BEAUTIFUL WELLNESS, LLC
12970 Ormond Way
King George, VA 22485
Phone: 540-775-3986, 540-226-1114

Misha Thomas
OPTIMAL HEALTH DIMENSIONS
3930 Pender Dr., ste. 280
Fairfax, VA 22030
Phone: 703-359-9300 Fax: 703-359-7814

Teresa Yvonne Owens
NATURAL HORIZON'S WELLNESS CENTERS
11230 Waples Mill Rd., suite 125
Fairfax , VA 22030

Judith M. Toscano ND, MT
THE WELLNESS COTTAGE
104 Via Ave. PO Box 1436
Stuart, VA 24171
Phone: 276-694-3650

Iris F. Carlo
OPTIMAL HEALTH DIMENSIONS
3930 Pender Dr., ste. 260
Fairfax, VA 22030
Phone: 703-359-9300 Fax: 703-359-7814

Wah-Keng Wu
VITALITY CLEANSING, LLC
44121 Harry Byrd Highway, suite 115
Ashburn, VA 20147
Phone: 703-271-0491

Emmanuel Kwame Asenso ND, NP
HEALTH TALK, INC.
6130 Wicklow Dr.
Burke, VA 22015
Phone: 703-822-7471 / 703-599-9035

Veronica Sam
OPTIMAL HEALTH DIMENSIONS
3930 Pender Dr., ste. 280
Fairfax, VA 22030
Phone: 703-359-9300 Fax: 703-359-7814

Marie Carol Alphonse
HOLISTIC COLON HYDROTHERAPY CENTER, LLC
14 Riggs Road
Fredericksburg, VA 22405
Phone: 540-479-6828 Fax: 540-479-6828

Vermont

Judy Plantin Charles
ALTERNATIVE THERAPEUTIC CENTER
25 Morgan Parkway
Williston, VT 05495
Phone: 802-879-0945

Washington

Dorothy Croft
DAYSPRING CLEANSING SPA
1703 Texas St.
Bellingham, WA 98229
Phone: 360-961-6400

Pamela Diane McCann
PJ'S ANGELIC RESOURCES
1639 S. 310th St., Ste. A
Federal Way , WA 98003
Phone: 253-941-5200

Bozena Nowicka
EUROPEAN REJUVENATION CENTER
4315 Factoria Blvd. SE, Suite #A
Bellevue, WA 98006
Phone: 425-746-6100

Danielle D. Huff
INTERNAL HARMONY
1333 Lincoln St., ste.#2
Bellingham , WA 98229
Phone: 360-734-1099

Wendy L. Stanger
STANGER MASSAGE AND HEALTH CENTER
1679 Grant Rd.
E. Wenatchee, WA 98802
Phone: 509-886-8592 Fax: 509-886-3612

ETERNA HOLISTIC THERAPIES
2825 80th Ave., SE., Suite 202
Mercer Island, WA 98040
Phone: 206-683-9552

Shannon C. Wallace
INTERNAL HARMONY
1333 Lincoln St, Suite 2
Bellingham, WA 98229
Phone: 360-734-1099

Wisconsin

Cecelia Senn
ANGELIC LIGHT HEALING CENTER
E5595 State Hwy. 82
Uiroqua, WI 54665
Phone: 608-299-0699

Jeffrey G. Karls
FOUNTAIN OF YOUTH - NATURAL HEALTH
6502 Normandy Lane
Madison, WI 53719
Phone: 608-516-4483 Fax: 608-826-9081

Laurean Millonzi RMT
DAY SPRING
N 88 W 16691 Appleton Ave
Menomonee Falls, WI 53051
Phone: 262-251-1697 Fax: 414-803-4783

Kristina M. Amelong
OPTIMAL HEALTH CENTER
3714 Atwood Ave.
Madison, WI 53714
Phone: 608-242-0200

Laura Potter
HEALTH NATURALLY, LLC
212 Green Bay Rd., Ste 102
Thiensville, WI 53092
Phone: 262-242-6550 Fax: 262-242-6575

Emily Brossette
THE BODYWORX CLINIC
W236S7050 Big Bend Drive, suite 5
Big Bend, WI 53103
Phone: 262-436-1360

Jacqueline Shoebridge
GENTLE WATERS
1111 15th Ave.
Bloomer, WI 54724
Phone: 715-933-1482
Email: shoe@bloomer.net
Cert. Level: Foundation

Jane M. Guyette
INNER AWAKENING HEALING CENTER
209 E. River Dr.
DePere, WI 54115
Phone: 209-985-2691

Mary S. Adams
NATURAL HEALTH MINISTRIES, INC.
23 South Main St., Suite 1
Hartford, WI 53027
Phone: 262-670-0184 Fax: 262-670-1059

Alice M. Miller
N2678 Manley Rd
Hortonville, WI 54944
Phone: 920-779-6041

Gale A. Ulbert
9223 74th St.
Kenosha, WI 53142
Phone: 262-705-6416 Fax: 262-942-6172

Crystel Lyons
ALMOST EDEN HOME SPA
7709-12th St.
Somers, WI 53171
Phone: 262-859-2121 Fax: 262-859-0369

West Virginia

Challen W. Waychoff N.D.
HEAVENLY WATER
1061 Market St.
Wheeling, WV 26003
Phone: 304-230-9283

Wyoming

Torill S. Morton
WARM RIVER HEALTH SOLUTIONS
906 Sonata Lane
Cheyenne, WY 82007
Phone: 307-760-9046

Sara Atkins
THE WHITE ROOMS - YORKSHIRE
203 Broaogate Lane, Horsforth
Leeds, West Yorkshire LS18 5BS
 United Kingdom
Phone: 0784-924-9247   ?

Michelle Lorraine Clark
BODY & SOUL ZONE
5A New Broadway
Ealing Broadway, London W5 5AW
 United Kingdom
Phone: 0208 810 1674

Sylvia Orsi
AQUA DI AQUA
18 East Barnet Road
New Barnet, Herts EN4 8RW
 United Kingdom
Phone: 0114320 8441 4432

Susie McFarlane
CHAMPNEYS FOREST MERE
Champneys Forest Mere
Lip Hook, Hampshire GU307JQ
 United Kingdom
Phone: 00441428726013

A Pearson
VEVAQUA COLONIC HYDROTHERAPY
8 Sun Street
Baldock, Hertfordshire, England SG7 6QA
 United Kingdom
Phone: 44 (0) 1462 490591

C Pearson
VEVAQUA COLONIC HYDROTHERAPY
8 Sun Street
Baldock, Hertfordshire, England SG7 6QA
 United Kingdom
Phone: 44 (0) 1462 490591

Sophie Weston
THE BEECHWOOD CLINIC
41 Hills Road
Cambridge, CB2 1NT
 United Kingdom
Phone: 01223 262013

Amanda Griggs
BALANCE THE CLINIC
250 Kings Rd.
Chelsea, London, England SW3 5UE
 United Kingdom
Phone: 00442075650333 Fax: 00442073515746

Emily Jane Bailey
CHIC HAIR & BEAUTY GROUP
4 Heathfield Road, Wigston
Leicester, LE18 1JR
 United Kingdom
Phone: 011-44-116-288-7433 or 011-44-116-251-8619

Suzanne Winfield
THE BRITISH SCHOOL OF COLON HYDROTHERAPY
Stoodley Hunting Lodge, Stoodley Lane
Eastwood, Todmorden, West Yorkshire OL146HA
 United Kingdom
Phone: 44 1 706 818332 Fax: 01706521720

Michelle Geraghty
ETERNAL BEING
54, London Road, Oadby
Leicester, England LE2 5DH
 United Kingdom
Phone: 0116 2717183

Shemila A. Tharani
BODY VIBRANT COLON HYDROTERAPY LIFE STORY
THERAPEUTIC CENTRE
17 Eldon Square
Reading, Berkshire RG14DP
 United Kingdom
Phone: 01189580806

Deborah Tennant BSc (Hons)
FRESH AS A DAISY (COLON CARE)
Fort Horsted Business Centre
Chatham, Kent, England ME4 6HZ
 United Kingdom

Linda Ternent
CASTLE STREET CLINIC
36-37 Castle Street (also have London Address)
Guildford, Surrey, England GU1 3UQ
 United Kingdom

Carole Holmback
THE KI CLINIC
The Old Stables
Hexham, Northunberland NE46 1XD
 United Kingdom
Phone: 01 434 6081 89

Jayne Timmins
HYDRO CLEANSE DETOXIFICATION &
REJUVENATION CLINIC
36 a
The Tything, Worcestershire WR1 1JL
 United Kingdom
Phone: 01905 2882 . √

Dharini Odedra
THE D-TOX CLINIC
1 Goldhill Rd.
Leicester, LE79RN
 United Kingdom
Phone: 07940346200

Marlin V. Armstrong
HEAVENLY SPA
1 Chilworth Mews
London, W2 3RG
 United Kingdom
Phone: 020 7298 3820 Fax: 020 7298 3830

Edwige Cabanetos
4 BALANCE & HEALTH
Flat 9-31 Calvin Street
London, England E1 6NW
 United Kingdom
Phone: 0207 247 7742 or 0795 875 5536

Velile S. Ndebele
AQUALIBRIA
1 Harley Street
London, England W1G 9QD
 United Kingdom
Phone: 44-0-800-612-9481

Julia A. Fionda
AQUA DI AQUA
18 East Barnet Road
New Barnet, Herts EN4 8RW
 United Kingdom
Phone: 0114320 8441 4432

Louise Knecht
SUNSHINE COLONICS
21, Ford Road
Old Woking, England GU229HJ
 United Kingdom

Richard Armstrong
HEAVENLY SPA
1 Chilworth Mews
London, W2 3RG
 United Kingdom
Phone: 020 7298 3820 Fax: 020 7298 3830

Reena Patel
PURE CLEANSE LTD BASED IN SANDRIDGE SURGERY
Sandridge
St. Albans, Hertfordshire, England AL4 9DB
 United Kingdom
Phone: 44-0-7939-559838

Sharon Fisher
ADVANCED DERMACARE
95, Trentham Rd.
Stoke on Trent, Staffordshire ST34EG
 United Kingdom
Phone: 01782313737

Catherine Marie Thompson
THE DETOX SHOP/ALBANY HEALTH CLINIC
1, Broomfield Road, Earlsdon Coventry
West Midlands, England CV5 6JW
 United Kingdom
Phone: 0044-247-671-2790

Relevant Websites

**Association of Registered
Colon Hydrotherapists**
www.colonic-association.org

**International Association and Register of Integrative
Colon Therapists and Trainers**
www.colonic-association.net

International Association for Hydrotherapy
www.i-act.org

The Art of Health
www.theartofhealth.us/pages/colonhydrotherapy.html

Colonic Network
http://www.colonic.net

National Board for Colon Hydrotherapy
http://www.nbcht.org

Wellness Within
http://wellnesswithinwi.com

The Natural Path Alternative
http://www.healthycleansing.com/

While it is highly recommended that you read the entire text to understand how the colon functions in the human gastrointestinal tract, and how colonics can enhance that functioning, the following are some of the most commonly asked questions on this topic.

What exactly is colonic hydrotherapy?

You may also see the terms colonic irrigation, high colonic, or colonic lavage to describe this procedure. Using repeated flushing with water, the therapy effectively cleanses the colon of accumulated waste.

What is the colon?

Also referred to as the large intestine or bowel, the colon is a five-foot-long tubular passage at the end of the human digestive tract. It measures roughly 2.5 inches (6.35 cm) in diameter.

The colon's function is to eliminate waste material from the body and conserve water. The bacteria in the colon synthesizes nutrients from the food we eat.

Why do people opt to undergo colon cleansing procedures?

Adherents of colon cleansing believe that our modern lifestyle, which couples high stress levels with a poor diet, is not optimum for efficient digestive performance.

If the colon cannot clear out all the waste material it processes, inflammation, infection, and a host of problems from simple constipation to colorectal cancer have a greater chance of becoming established in the bowel.

Colon cleansing supports the natural function of the bowel and promotes overall good health.

Won't an enema or laxative do the same thing?

Enemas will effectively empty the last 8-12 inches of the colon called the rectum. Laxatives do the same thing, and are useful for alleviating temporary constipation.

Hydrotherapy, however, reaches all areas of the bowel, strengthening the muscles in the process, and promoting more regular, natural bowel movements.

Are there any added benefits to having a colonic?

Yes. You will be working with a trained therapist for 45 minutes to an hour. During that time, you will discuss your diet and lifestyle, exploring other adjustments you can make to support healthy bowel function.

While a colonic treatment does serve specifically to thoroughly empty the bowel of waste, the true goal of the treatment is a bettering of your total health profile.

Is the colonic procedure painful?

On rare occasions people do experience a mild cramping during a colonic. These episodes pass quickly, and are not difficult to tolerate.

Therapists are trained to put their clients at ease, and ready to answer any questions or concerns. Mention any discomfort immediately.

Isn't a colonic just a little too embarrassing?

The procedure is conducted in a private room with a trained therapist whose job is not only to administer the therapy, but to put you at ease and to preserve your dignity.

You will be covered at all times, and the parts of the procedure people dread most, including any odor, do not occur because the colonic apparatus is a closed system.

What should I do to get ready for a colonic irrigation session?

Eat or drink very lightly a couple of hours before the procedure. There is no need to fast, or to make any major adjustments in your normal routine.

Should I do anything special after the procedure is over?

Over the course of a few hours, you may have more bowel movements, but these are not uncomfortable or uncontrollable in terms of urgency. Just carry on with your normal routine.

Is there any danger involved in colonic hydrotherapy?

When working with a trained therapist in a professional environment where the equipment is properly cleaned and sterilized, there is virtually no danger to this therapy whatsoever.

I've heard getting colonics is habit forming. Is this true?

This is a myth. The goal of the therapy is a colon that functions properly. After the procedure, it may take a while for the next bowel movement to occur, which leads some people to think they have become dependent on the procedure to eliminate.

With dietary and lifestyle changes to support colon health, however, better regularity of function is almost assured.

Will colonic hydrotherapy lead to constipation or diarrhea?

Typically after a colonic session there will be a delay before the next bowel movement. When it does occur, the stool is generally somewhat larger and easier to move. Any instance of diarrhea is very rare and short-lived.

I have been suffering from constipation. Will colonic cleansing help?

In order for your colon to function properly, you must have a good balance of nutrition and hydration, physical exercise, and emotional well-being. The colonic will clear out the bowel sufficiently to allow the other factors to be adjusted in a much more physically comfortable state.

I've read that colonics get rid of all the beneficial intestinal bacteria and rob the system of nutrients. Is any of that true?

The bacteria your intestine needs to function can only grow in a balanced environment. They live on the wall of the colon and are not removed during colonic hydrotherapy.

If there is reason to believe that the bacteria in your bowel is out of balance, the therapist may implant a post-treatment probiotic or suggest that you begin a course of probiotic treatment to correct the issue.

Does colon cleansing benefit the immune system?

Recent studies completed in Europe have found that as much as 80% of the immune tissue in the human body resides in the intestines.

Since hydrotherapy promotes a healthy colon and works to reduce inflammation, it also serves to protect the immune function of the bowel.

How much time should I set aside for the procedure?

On your first visit with a therapist, 15-30 minutes will be taken up filling out forms and discussing your medical history. After that, the duration of the treatment varies by individual, but typically takes about 34 minutes. For your first appointment, set aside at least two hours.

Is it alright to eat after a colonic?

Have a regular meal at the time you normally eat. Don't over eat, and try to consume something that is both gentle and nourishing to your system.

I have problem skin. Will colon cleansing help?

Since your skin is also an important organ for the elimination of waste, it stands to reason that toxicity anywhere in the system will cause the skin to suffer. In many cases, clients find that colon cleansing is very beneficial to their problem skin.

How many colon cleansing treatments will I need?

Although most people feel definite improvement in their sense of wellbeing after a single treatment, changes in diet and lifestyle are necessary to really achieve the goal of a healthy digestive system.

If you have a long-standing condition, it's difficult to assess how many treatments will be required. If you opt for a maintenance program of therapy, the period in between session will grow longer as your bowel health optimizes.

Will colon cleansing help me to lose weight?

You will definitely feel lighter after a colonic treatment. There may be some weight loss, but the real improvement will be evident when you begin to take in more fiber, increase your level of exercise, and drink more water.

While these things support good bowel function, they also contribute to safe and permanent weight loss.

Should colonics be administered during pregnancy?

Typically colonics should not be administered during pregnancy unless the procedure is performed by a qualified medical practitioner.

How soon after giving birth can I have a colonic?

Wait 10-12 weeks after a normal childbirth to have a colonic; longer if the birth was difficult or a C-Section was required. The body needs a chance to fully recover, and any stitches must be healed completely. Nursing mothers can have colonics with no ill effects to themselves or to their child.

Glossary

A

abdomen - On the human body, the area located between the chest and the hips. Internally, this area contains the stomach, small and large intestines, liver, gallbladder, pancreas, and spleen.

absorption - The process by which the small intestine draws nutrients from food into the body's cells.

anemia - A disorder of the blood marked by a deficiency in red blood cells.

anus - The opening at the end of the human digestive tract through which the waste contents of the bowel exit the body.

ascending colon - The portion of the colon located on the right side of the body.

B

barium - A chalk-like liquid used as a coating for the inside of organs to make them more visible on X-rays.

bile - This fluid, produced by the liver and stored in the gallbladder, breaks down fats and assists in removing wastes from the body.

bloating - A feeling of fullness or actual swelling of the abdomen often present after meals.

bowel - An alternative word for the large intestine or colon.

bowel movement - The series of muscular contractions that leads to the elimination of wastes from the body through the rectum and anus.

C

cecum - The first section of the large intestine.

celiac disease - A disease caused by a reaction of the human immune system to the protein gluten found in grains like wheat, rye, and barley among other foods. The small intestine is damaged and cannot properly absorb nutrients, leading to diarrhea, anemia, and weight loss.

colic - Abdominal pain caused by muscle spasm in the intestines.

colitis - An irritation of the colon.

colon - The proper term for the large intestine or bowel.

colonoscopy - A procedure that allows the entire length of the colon to be viewed for diagnostic purposes and the removal or biopsy of any abnormal growths or polyps.

colorectal cancer - Any cancer that is present in either the colon or the rectum.

colon cleansing - Any one of several alternative therapies that strive to remove toxins and accumulated waste from the colon for the purpose of promoting proper functioning while detoxifying the system and preventing inflammation.

colostomy - An operation whereby stool leaves the body via an alternative route when the rectum has either been removed or when the area requires healing after surgery. A colostomy may be a temporary or permanent measure.

constipation - Difficulty emptying the bowels due to a hardening of the feces. Typically said to exist when there are fewer than three bowel movements per week.

Crohn's disease - A chronic inflammatory bowel disease of the lower small intestine.

D

defecation - The removal of the waste contents of the bowel through the rectum and anus.

dehydration - A loss of fluids in the body that can be attributed to many factors including diarrhea.

descending colon - That portion of the colon on the left side of the abdomen in which stool is stored prior to defecation.

digestion - The process by which the body breaks down food and extracts nutrients to create energy, facility growth, and repair cells.

digestive tract - Organs in the body that are responsible for food digestion. This tract starts at the mouth and is comprised of the salivary glands, esophagus, stomach, pancreas, liver, gallbladder, small intestine, and large intestine.

diverticulitis - A condition of the colon in which small pouches become infected and irritated.

duodenum - The first section of the small intestine.

E

esophagus - The organ of the digestive tract that connects the mouth to the stomach.

F

feces - Solid waste matter eliminated from the body through the rectum during bowel movements.

fiber - Plant matter obtained in food that aids digestion by softening the stool for easier passage out of the body.

flatulence - Excessive gas that builds up in the stomach or intestines that may also cause bloating.

G

gallbladder - The organ in the digestive system that stores bile produced by the liver and delivers it to the small intestine to assist in fat digestion.

gas - Air that accumulates as part of the normal breakdown of food in digestion. It is passed from the body through either the rectum or the mouth.

gastric - Of our related to the stomach.

gluten - A protein found in wheat, rye, barley, and oats to which many people have a dietary sensitivity.

H

hemorrhoids - Swollen blood vessels in or adjacent to the anus that cause symptoms including itching, pain, and occasional bleeding.

I

ileum - The lower end of the small intestine.

J

jejunum - The middle section of the small intestine lying between the duodenum and the ileum.

L

large intestine - That portion of the intestine between the cecum and the rectum.

lavage - A cleansing of the stomach or colon by using special drinks and/or enemas.

laxative - A medication for the relief of constipation.

liver - The largest of the bodily organs charged with the function of producing bile, converting food to energy, and cleaning out poisons and alcohol from the blood.

M

malabsorption syndrome - Any condition that causes the small intestine to be unable to absorb nutrients from foods.

mucus - A thick substance with the consistency of jelly produced by the intestines and other bodily organs. Mucus serves to coat and protect the lining of an organ and in the large intestine and rectum facilitates the easy passage of stool.

P

pancreas - A gland in the digestive system that produces enzymes and the hormone insulin.

perforation - A hole created in the wall of an organ as a consequence of disease or medical error.

peristalsis - The motion of the muscles in the gastrointestinal tract that creates waves that move food and liquid down the digestive course.

pharynx - The area behind the mouth through which food passes on the way to the esophagus and through which air passes from the nose and mouth to the larynx.

polyp - A bulb-like mass of cells attached to a stalk found on the surface or in the inner lining of an organ.

R

rectum - The lower end of the large intestine or colon that leads to the anus.

S

sigmoid colon - The lower part of the colon that connects to, and thus empties into the rectum.

sigmoidoscopy - A diagnostic procedure that allows for the visual examination of the lower portions of the colon.

small intestine - The portion of the digestive system lying between the stomach and the large intestine where the bulk of digestion and nutrient absorption occurs.

stomach - The digestive organ lying between the esophagus and the small intestine where the digestion of protein starts to occur.

stool - Undigested foods and associated matter included mucus, bacteria, and dead cells that are eliminated from the body as solid wastes through the rectum.

T

transverse colon - That part of the colon which cross the abdomen from right to left.

U

ulcerative colitis - A disease of the colon and rectum in which open ulcers and adjacent irritations form on the inner lining of both sections of the digestive tract.

Index

autoimmune disorders, 69

bacteria, 20, 31, 32, 36, 43, 47, 177, 181, 192

bowel function, 39, 47, 64, 66, 80, 178, 183

Caffeine, 63

chronic fatigue, 17, 43, 44

closed-system colonic treatment, 49

colon cleansing, 3, 15, 16, 35, 36, 59, 60, 65, 67, 178, 181, 182, 183, 187

colonic hydrotherapy, 2, 3, 13, 36, 42, 47, 59, 69, 75, 80, 81, 177, 180, 181

colonic therapy, 49, 53

Colonoscopy, 28, 69, 70, 71

Dairy, 64

digestive system, 1, 2, 3, 17, 36, 42, 45, 69, 183, 189, 190, 191

digestive tract, 2, 21, 44, 47, 64, 73, 74, 79, 177, 185, 188, 192

Enema, 54

exercise, 24, 28, 32, 75, 77, 78, 181, 183

fats, 31, 43, 66, 185

fiber, 24, 25, 60, 61, 62, 66, 67, 74, 183, 188

fish, 66

food dyes, 1

genetically modified, 1, 32

GI tract, 27, 75

gluten, 1, 30, 32, 66, 186, 189

grain, 1, 66

growth hormones, 1

hydration, 39, 64, 181

immune system, 17, 27, 42, 43, 45, 46, 181, 186

Inflammation, 45

joint pain, 17, 43

laxatives, 15, 16, 53, 54, 55

Leaky Gut Syndrome, 41, 42

LIBBE system, 51

maltodextrins, 74

massage therapy, 49

Open Colonic System, 51

pharmaceuticals, 1, 60

Polyps, 22, 70

preservatives, 1, 59, 63

Processed foods, 63

processed sugars, 1

proteins, 43, 47

psyllium, 61

rectum, 20, 21, 28, 49, 50, 51, 70, 178, 186, 187, 188, 189, 190, 191, 192

sigmoidoscopy, 11, 23, 28, 70, 71, 191

skin rashes, 43

sodium, 1

speculum, 49, 50

stress, 17, 33, 45, 74, 76, 178

The Gerson Therapy, 65

toxic chemicals, 1

toxins, 2, 3, 11, 41, 43, 45, 46, 62, 73, 74, 75, 76, 79, 187

whole grains, 66

Wood's Gravity method, 50

yeast, 43, 45

Yoga, 78

zinc, 45

Printed in Great Britain
by Amazon

34960083R00109